T0243085

Evaluation for a Caring Society

A volume in
Evaluation and Society
Jennifer C. Greene and Stewart I. Donaldson, *Series Editors*

Evaluation for a Caring Society

edited by

Merel Visse

University of Humanistic Studies

Tineke A. Abma

VU University Medical Center

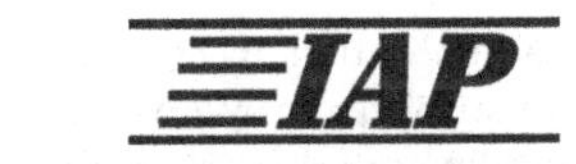

INFORMATION AGE PUBLISHING, INC.
Charlotte, NC • www.infoagepub.com

Library of Congress Cataloging-in-Publication Data

A CIP record for this book is available from the Library of Congress
http://www.loc.gov

ISBN: 978-1-64113-163-6 (Paperback)
978-1-64113-164-3 (Hardcover)
978-1-64113-165-0 (ebook)

Printed in the United States of America

CONTENTS

PART II

DEMOCRATIC EVALUATION FOR A CARING SOCIETY

PART III

ETHICS AND EVALUATION FOR A CARING SOCIETY

PART IV

RESPONSIVE EVALUATION FOR A CARING SOCIETY

FOREWORD

More than a half-century ago, C. Wright Mills criticized what he called abstracted empiricism in sociology, an approach that fetishized facts and evidence, equated empiricism with science, and advocated political disengagement. He also called for the development of the sociological imagination that makes possible the recognition of a relationship between private troubles and public issues. Today, in the broad and varied field of evaluation practice, Mills' concerns remain salient. The field is alarmed at the excessive emphasis on evidence-based best practices and at efforts to assign the highest value to empirical evidence gathered in an apolitical, technical fashion. Likewise, as many authors of this volume make clear, the growing concern with a caring and relational perspective on the aims and conduct of evaluation draws attention to how private woes evident in the context of the personal and biographical are to be interrelated with the sociological and political realm of public issues.

This book explores the relationship between evaluation as a professional practice and care (a particular type of concern for others) as well as caring (the act of attending to others in a particular way). On the one hand, care/caring might be reasonably thought of as an ethic for evaluation practice. It might be sensibly seen most poignantly as a relational ethic that governs the personal sphere, a means of guiding the various kinds of interpersonal and micropolitical interactions that professionals have with individuals they encounter in the course of professional work. It might be regarded as a companion to an ethic of justice that guides thinking and acting around issues

Evaluation for a Caring Society, pages vii–ix

in the macropolitical sphere surrounding how the profession promotes the public good for all citizens.

In this volume, however, I believe the editors are suggesting that care should be promoted not as an ethic but as an ethos for the professional practice of evaluation. This seems especially evident in the concluding synthesis chapter. An ethos refers to a group's distinguishing moral character and shared fundamental identity. It encompasses the professional group's motives, values, ways of reasoning, goals, aspirations, and, even, anxieties. An ethos more so than any set of ethical principles guides the interactions a professional has with those he or she serves.

References throughout this volume to care as a moral-political-epistemological practice (a disposition, a set of understandings, as well as a way of reasoning and acting) suggest this idea of a particular evaluation ethos. Evaluation is a social practice concerned with public issues most obviously manifest in private troubles with programs and policies in immigration, health care, education, social services, housing, and so on. A student of color experiences discrimination in a public school classroom in the United States; the evaluator is concerned not only with that child's experience but with the larger public, political issue of an achievement gap in public education between white students and students of color. An ethos of care in evaluation guides behavior at these two levels of action. At one level is the evaluator's immediately responsive and interpersonal encounter with the personal troubles of social actors, most visible, as Mills originally pointed out, in an individual's biography and in those social settings directly open to the individual's lived experience. A contemporary example is the evaluator who listens attentively, empathetically, and with care to the experience of an undocumented child of immigrant workers now enrolled in a college in the United States who is deeply worried he will be deported because the President of the United States is threatening to rescind a deferral program originally protecting this individual. At another level, the sociological and political level, the evaluator operates at what Mills called the arena of public issues where immediate personal troubles are seen not only as problems encountered by individuals but as the result of structural and political arrangements in society. Thus, the counterpart to the personal story is that the evaluator must be aware of and attentive to the fact that the lives of approximately 750,000 undocumented immigrants will be affected by the President's decision that is grounded in his ideological position on the issue of immigration. In the view of the editors of this volume, evaluation for a caring society is thought to operate at both levels.

Whether an ethos for evaluation wherein (in the words of the editors of this volume) "care is at the center of critically and responsively examining societal challenges and questions" and whereby evaluation promotes a caring society can be more fully articulated remains to be seen. But the present volume is certainly a strong step forward in that direction.

—Thomas A. Schwandt
Professor Emeritus
University of Illinois at Urbana-Champaign

FOREWORD

Evaluation and care are mutually related. As any practice, evaluation should be performed in an attentive and responsible way, showing a caring attitude. Thus, evaluation requires care. Care as a human activity should be responsive to the needs of those cared for, which asks for continuously checking the impact of one's actions. Consequently, care implies an element of evaluation. The intricate relationship between evaluation and care is hardly addressed by evaluators or caregivers. This book fills a gap, as it focuses on the relationship between evaluation and care and provides a multitude of examples of evaluation as a caring practice.

Why is the relationship between evaluation and care often overlooked? The importance of care to evaluation, and of evaluation to care, resembles the importance of water to fishes. As their natural habitat, water is not noticed by its inhabitants. It is not until the water dries down or becomes polluted, that the fishes become painfully aware of its crucial role in their existence. If they are lucky, they can escape to find fresh water, after which the awareness of the importance of it will feed away. Evaluators and caregivers also tend to forget the close relationship between evaluation and care, and its relevance to their practices. The authors in this book reflect on this relationship, and thus help the reader to become aware of aspects of their work which are normally not visible, and provide perspectives which may help to nurture these elements, and make their work better.

The mutual relationship between evaluation and care not only means that both refer to each other. Evaluation and care also share a common orientation, as they are both driven by values. The word evaluation already

Evaluation for a Caring Society, pages xi–xiii

indicates that values are at stake. An evaluation of a practice means to investigate whether the practice realizes the values which are relevant for and constitutive of that practice. Care also refers to values. In her theoretical analysis of care, referred to in many contributions to this book, Joan Tronto elucidates five core values: attentiveness, responsibility, competence, responsiveness and solidarity. According to her, these values are not general principles, guiding action from outside; they are virtues, embodied in the practice of caregivers. Thus, values are not external rules of conduct which are to be obeyed, but internal dispositions, acquired through and realized in the practice of care.

The intricate relationship between evaluation and care, and their orientation on values embodied in practice, sheds new light on current evaluation procedures, for instance the evaluation of scientific research. One may question whether standard evaluation protocols, focusing on output in terms of number of articles, actually investigate whether a scientist contributes to the realization of scientific values. The plea for taking into account social impact as an indicator of scientific quality refers to other parameters, and makes values explicit, as social impact is also denominated as social value. Yet, also the focus on social impact should be critically assessed. Often, this is interpreted as economic value. Scientists, however, can add value in other ways than developing products which are profitable. Products of medical science, such as medical technologies, should be investigated for their value for patients and other stakeholders. Do they meet the needs of vulnerable people? Do they support the process of care, and foster and embody core values like attentiveness and responsibility? These are crucial questions, as medical science ultimately aims at making the lives of patients better. Likewise, others scientific practices should be evaluated from the perspective of their contribution to the improvement of human life, including its natural and social environment.

The growing attention for research integrity is another example of both the importance of values in scientific practice, and the need to interpret these values in terms of care. The importance of research integrity is visible in the denunciation of fraud and fabrication of data and the retraction of articles when such actions are discovered. These actions clearly go against core values in science, like truth and reliability. Yet, it can be argued that being a good scientist requires not just compliance with rules which forbid such actions. Honesty and trustworthiness are virtues that should be embodied in everyday scientific practice, for instance in collaborating with colleagues, performing reviews, and approaching respondents. Thus, the evaluation of science from the perspective of research integrity should focus on investigating whether the practice of science is a practice of care.

This book provides excellent examples of evaluation of social practices from the perspective of care. Yet, it takes one step further. The aim is to shed light on evaluation itself as a practice of care. This is relevant in at least three ways. In the first place, evaluators who take a caring stance are motivated by concrete experiences of social needs and lived problems. They are touched by people, individually and as part of institutions, who are in need of care. In the second place, evaluators who are aware of the importance of a caring attitude, reflect on their relationship with practices which they are engaged with. Rather than taking a superior stance, and judging a practice from outside, they are sensitive to the effects of their work on the practice they investigate. In the third place, evaluators who see their work as a practice of care focus on engendering processes of mutual learning in and with the stakeholders involved. They see the importance of dialogues, not only between stakeholders, but also between investigators and the participants in the practice under study. From a perspective of care, these dialogues should focus on concrete experiences and result in new ways of dealing with felt needs.

Evaluation as a caring practice takes time. It requires investing in relationships, building a climate of trust, and responding when trust is under pressure. Caring implies getting to know people, listening to their daily concerns, and helping them to find ways of dealing with difficulties. Caring requires accurate timing: being present when needed, and offering support in a way which fits to the situation. Investing time by being present is not easy, in an era in which time is measured in minutes to be spent on performing tasks and in which the number of tasks tends to grow infinitely, like the number of emails in one's inbox. However, caring also creates time. The experience of mutual engagement in the process of care is a specific experience of time, which the hermeneutic philosopher Gadamer calls "fulfilled time." In contrast to the "empty time," which one experiences when having to perform meaningless activities, the experience of "fulfilled time" creates joy and happiness. It feels like it takes no time at all.

Reading a book like this volume certainly takes time. Instead of scanning abstracts, and looking for sentences which can be quoted in one's next article, the reader has to dive into the chapters and enter into their flow. This, however, will be rewarding, as the reader gradually will come to share the enthusiasm of the authors, and be enriched by their insights. In this way, the book can serve as an antidote to the present-day haste in social practices, and contribute, in form and content, to developing an evaluation practice which may foster a caring society.

—Guy Widdershoven
Professor of Philosophy and Ethics of Medicine
Head of the Department of Medical Humanities
VU University Medical Center, VU University Amsterdam.

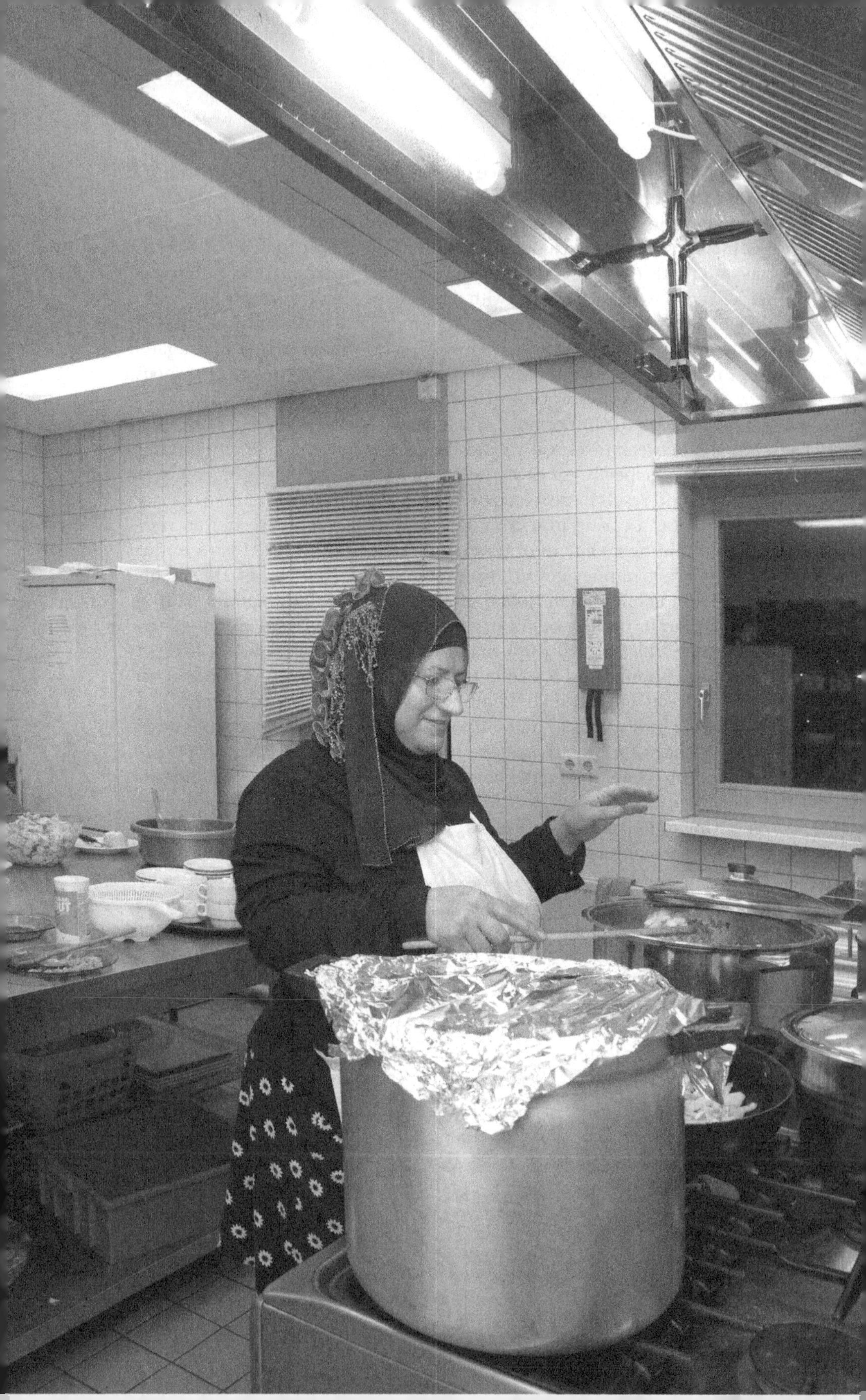

ACKNOWLEDGMENTS

The idea for this book emerged on two occasions. First in 2013, when one of us (Merel) met with Prof. Dr. Jennifer Greene at the yearly International Conference on Qualitative Inquiry in Illinois as part of her travel grant from the EMGO+/Amsterdam Public Health research institute. Jennifer informed whether we would be interested to develop a special Volume on humanization in evaluation. A year later, at the 2014 conference of the European Evaluation Association in Dublin, the three of us met again and our plans gradually grew. Together with professor dr. Anders Hanberger and Hannah Leyerzapf, we organized a session on Humanization in Evaluation. There, and the years following, we were delighted to continue our conversations with Jennifer and with professor Helen Simons, professor. dr. Bob Stake and many more. When one of us (Merel) moved to the Care Ethics group of the University of Humanistic Studies, the focus changed to the intersection of care ethics and evaluation studies.

There are so many inspiring evaluators and care ethicists and we would have loved to include the work of more of them, but we had to make (tough) choices. This book is not the end though. It's just the beginning of a quest for exploring the promises and pitfalls of evaluation as a praxis of care. Many people have helped us along the way and we are indebted to all of them, especially the authors of this Volume and Prof. dr. Thomas Schwandt and Prof. dr. Guy Widdershoven for the time they took too read the manuscript and write a foreword. We are indebted to Janine Schrijver, who generously shared her artistic work with us: the pictures of the Carefreestate that enliven this book and that spurred a conversation with Zaitone Osman, a

Evaluation for a Caring Society, pages xv–xvi

voice reflected in a poem. Our greatest thanks goes to the women of the pictures in this book: by sharing their stories they provide us with a glimpse into the everyday reality of care. Our thanks also go to our colleagues at the Care Ethics Group in Utrecht and the Medical Humanities Department, VU University medical center in Amsterdam.

Our greatest gratitude and appreciation goes to Jennifer Greene. It is because of her inspiration, warmth, support and wisdom that this book has become a reality.

—Dr. Merel Visse
Prof. dr. Tineke Abma

INTRODUCTION

Merel Visse
University of Humanistic Studies

Tineke Abma
VU University Medical Center

I am going to learn to make bread tomorrow. So you may imagine me with my sleeves rolled up, mixing flour, milk, salaratus, etc., with a great deal of grace. I advise you if you don't know how to make the staff of life to learn with dispatch. I think I could keep house very comfortably if I knew how to cook. But as long as I don't, my knowledge of housekeeping is about of as much use as faith without works, which you know we are told is dead.

—Emily Dickinson to Abiah Root, September 25, 1845

What happens when domestic bliss does not create bliss? Laura tries to bake a cake. She cracks an egg. The cracking egg becomes a common gesture throughout the film [The Hours, dir. By S. Daldry, 2002], *connecting the domestic labor of women over time. To bake a cake ought to be a happy activity, a labor of love. Instead, the film reveals a sense of oppression that lingers in the very act of breaking eggs. Not only do such objects not make you happy; they embody a feeling of disappointment. The bowl in which you crack your eggs waits for you. You can feel the pressure of its wait. The empty bowl feels like an accusation.*

—Sara Ahmet, on the film *The Hours*, 2017, p. 63

Evaluation for a Caring Society, pages 1–15

NURTURING A CARING SOCIETY

This book explores the intersection of evaluation studies and care ethics in contemporary Western societies. In all societies and institutions, large and small, we find forces that can strengthen or destroy their fabric. One new regulation, law, or policy can impact the lives of many who find themselves in precarious positions. Think, for example, about health care reform and migrant policies in various Western countries and their effects on the everyday lives of millions of people. Policies, programs, and those who execute them can threaten the daily routines of our lives, and we can respond by withdrawing or freezing, doing nothing and thinking it will pass. Or we can respond with resistance, anger, and sometimes much worse, like the shootings in several American cities.

This may sound like an overly dramatic opening to a book about evaluation and care, but in our work as evaluators, we have encountered similar responses to changes in society. Take, for example the response of a nurse to the announcement of a new accountability policy in elderly care: "They don't trust me. I'll quit." This nurse did not find it comforting that the managers who announced this policy change felt as stuck as he did, forced by changes in regulations beyond their control. In every situation where tensions grow and are not resolved, people are inclined to protect themselves ("I'll quit") and increase control (new rules), instead of exercising care and creativity. They abandon their connections not only with others but also with themselves.

We would like to change that and accordingly recall what women have known for ages and Rebecca Solnit (2017, p. 18) recently articulated powerfully: the power of interconnectedness and gathering for solidarity, support, and advice. Think of the mother with a child at her breast. In case of danger, she cannot simply run away or pick arms and go to war. She is involved in survival and nurturing activities to protect herself and her offspring and to promote safety in an environment characterized by uncertainty and instability. This is why the presence of a life-sustaining web (Fisher & Tronto, 1990, p. 40) is central to care ethicists. They view people as part of such webs that support them in living their lives as well as possible (Fisher & Tronto, 1990, p. 40). This ethical notion of care prompts our exploration of how we can contribute to (and think about) a caring society. Let us then begin with our own practice: the practice and theory of evaluation. We write this book for that reason: to integrate notions from care ethics into evaluation theory and practice in order to nurture a caring society.

Evaluators' task is to assess and understand the impact of policies and programs on people's lives. In our view, policy and program evaluation can and should advance humanization and care. The work of evaluators should create "ethical" spaces with a "temporary suspension of ethical assumptions" (Kushner, 2000, p. 151). This can promote trust and solidarity, prerequisites to recognizing the meaningfulness and humanity of everyday practices. However, evaluation is typically conducted in politicized contexts, with many competing sets of values and priorities, so a vision guiding the evaluation practice is needed. Care ethics can inspire such a vision.

Together with colleagues in the fields of evaluation studies and care ethics, we, in this book, invite you to learn about the possibilities and challenges of integrating evaluation studies and care ethics in the service of a caring society—a society with policies and programs that honor and respect people's vulnerability, precariousness, interdependencies, and needs. Including these human features in our evaluative and care ethical work weaves new threads into our work and, over time, our social fabric. We envision that this fabric will leave neoliberal views on humanity in the past and move toward a different but more realistic view that honors who we are.

In this book, we seek to address how we, as scholars in the evaluation and ethics field, can contribute to a society that honors care while acknowledging and respecting the realities of regulation and financial incentives that control the public sector. Connecting theoretical and empirical work from a rich variety of scholars and fields of inquiry, we gradually develop a view on evaluation as an approach to nurturing a caring society. This view and its implications for evaluation studies are presented in the last discussion chapter.

FROM EQUITY TO CARE

This book emerged from the 2014 conference of the European Evaluation Association in Dublin. At that conference, the notion of *equity* was prominent and debated widely. Equity was addressed in the context of programs and policies, with a special interest in approaches aimed fostering equity, such as equity-focused evaluation, democratic evaluation, and transdisciplinary evaluation. Fervent debates raged over formative and summative evaluations and the rights and obligations of evaluators while carrying out their studies, such as the right to set criteria in advance and do justice to those criteria. To our surprise, we noticed that the discourse was abstract and principled, relatively detached from the everyday complexities and practices of evaluation. The discussion focused on evaluations approached with pre-set criteria and the application of principles to particular cases to determine the effectiveness of an evaluation. The conversations at that conference assumed that issues of fairness and the rights and obligations of program and policy participants should be on the agenda and can be assessed impartially. This presumption resembles justice thinking as a rights-based moral theory, which emphasizes autonomy, equality, and the fair distribution of goods among as many as possible. In liberal and neoliberal climates, principles of justice are agreed upon by people assumed to be capable of agreeing or disagreeing with social arrangements. Not each and every citizen, though, is able to participate in rational deliberation as a free, equal agent (Held, 2015), nor can certain forms of injustice be articulated in the prevailing discourse.

However, in some evaluation studies, rules have been followed, but justice has not been done, especially with regards to the inclusion of multiple perspectives in particular situations. Evaluators such as Ernest House, Robert Stake, Egon Guba, Yvonna Lincoln, and Thomas Schwandt have long argued for a more situated, dialogical, practice-oriented view on evaluations to counter the use of explicated standards and allow space for context. Why then did equity still dominate the conference? Why did we notice a lack of care for particularity and contextuality? We wondered whether justice thinking in evaluation studies, accompanied by a discourse of preset criteria, equity, autonomy, rights, and obligations, could be opened up (again) to create space for the contextuality, relationality, and situatedness of people in evaluations.

A CALL TO CARE

We, therefore, aim to incorporate care ethics into the discussion on equity and justice in evaluation settings. Within the field of moral philosophy, care ethicists and theorists have extensively scrutinized theories on justice—not only as a theoretical field but also in the context of moral education and development. Care ethicists agree that care ethics began with the work of Carol Gilligan (1982). In her book *In a Different Voice*, Gilligan (1982) criticizes Kohlberg's notion that the highest form of moral development arises from impartial, abstract principles of justice and Kantian reasoning. She explains that the impartial justice model conflicts with other important elements in moral decision making, often emphasized by women, such as maintaining relationships despite divergent interests and desires, a commitment to meeting others' concrete needs, and needing certain feelings and emotions to understand a situation. To prevent an opposition between justice and care, Gilligan (1982) argues that justice should include care. Justice then becomes also constituted by care and the capacity to take care of and be attentive to others.

Care ethics, as an interdisciplinary field of study (Leget, van Nistelrooij, & Visse, 2017), regards people as "dependent upon one another for their survival, development and social functioning, and highlights the unchosen obligations we all have towards others by virtue of our interdependency" (Engster, 2007, p. 7)—unchosen and interdependent because we have lost control and do not have a complete understanding of the forces that influence our society, our institutions, our families, and sometimes even ourselves. To continue our lives and work, we pay attention to and care for and about others, systems, and their routines. We care in many different ways and in a variety of areas. Care is easily found in ordinary, personal settings regarded as relational in nature (Van Nistelrooij, 2014). A child cannot grow up without feeding from a parent; an adult cannot die with dignity without sincere support. During the rest of our lives, our house becomes a home because we care, we can have a meal when we are ill because someone cooks for us, and on Monday, our colleagues inquire after our weekend to reconnect and get back to work. Consequently, in contrast to justice thinking, care ethics does not only see people as reasoners but also recognizes that people cannot reach unambiguous agreement upon a single interpretation of principles. Principles and regulations are always open to multiple interpretations, especially when applied in real-life situations.

Some care ethicists see care as a normative concept (Barnes, 2012). As soon as we begin to think about care, we start to ponder what good care entails. Others see care as primarily descriptive (Kittay, 2015). Just as we don't say "good justice," we should not say "good care." The goodness of care is already part of its meaning (Kittay, 2015, p. 69). Despite these different views on the descriptive and normative nature of care, care theorists make it very clear that care is a *practice*. Care is more than *caring for*. It also includes *caring about* (Tronto, 1993). Caring for is an act; it refers to doing and acting, and is an important phase of care, requiring expertise and technical knowledge. However, equally important to good care are attentiveness to others' needs, acceptance of responsibility for others, and responsiveness to their changing needs and desires. Joan Tronto (2014) explicitly states that good care is linked to these moral virtues. Good care is always a two-way affair; it cannot be delivered in a paternalistic or parochial way. The receiver needs to be open to and responsive to the care given. Nel Noddings (2015) adds that care can be good only when the receiver acknowledges the care that is given. This requires that the care receiver, who is dependent on the caregiver, grant trust and authority to the caregiver (Tronto, 2014).

To us, care ethics generally moves from what is *just*, from rights and principles to *what matters* to people, to "assess the import of things for people," their evaluative judgements (Sayer, 2011, p. 6). It also moves from reason to perception and experience: putting *lived experience* in everyday situations at the center of attention (Laugier, 2014). Care ethics, however, is not solely concerned with eliciting and understanding lived experience in relational settings. It is a political and critical ethic focused on comprehending how society is constituted by people who relate to each other in situations both of peace and of conflict and tension. Care ethicists acknowledge that the people in a society are interdependent, fragile, vulnerable, and enmeshed in asymmetrical relationships and need to relate to each other in meaningful ways. Care ethicists acknowledge that we are *all* born in a state of dependency and alternately give and receive care throughout our lives. Thus, care is deeply political (Engster, 2007; Tronto, 2014; Visse, Abma, & Widdershoven, 2015). Care is not only about attending and supporting others' needs nor solely about giving and receiving care in personal realms. It is about much more than that.

Care is the fabric of our sociopolitical lives. Care plays a crucial role in the stability and growth of our institutions, policies, and programs. For example, health care and social policies often are aimed at prescribing who should care for whom and in what way. Care is not solely a personal undertaking but is also manifested in political institutions (Engster, 2007, p. 6). As political ethics, care ethics puts care at the center of thinking about society and democracy. Instead of taking the link between political liberalism and justice for granted, political care ethics questions core democratic values by introducing care as a way of repairing and maintaining our world, so we can live our lives as well as possible (Fisher & Tronto, 1990, p. 40). Political care ethics challenges the hierarchical, rational, and bureaucratic allocation of caring responsibilities to, for example, domestic migrant workers (Tronto, 2014). It critically scrutinizes and discusses the invisibility of care in our society. Care is too easily passed on by those in higher positions to those lower in the social hierarchy. *Privileged irresponsibility* is the term used to criticize these processes (Tronto, 1993). Care ethics thereby creates space for political dimensions of care, including power, and values such as solidarity.

Care, as a fabric, can hold together people in social practices but can also drive them apart, for example, in the case of care that is too protective or paternalistic. Too little or too much care builds or destroys a social practice. Care demands a "*middle way*": a balance to sustain life by engaging with others in joint social practices (Widdershoven & Huijer, 2001, p. 315). We seek appropriate responses to societal questions and challenges, such as how to care for the old, disabled, and chronically ill. Sometimes, we respond to emergency breakdowns of care, situations in which care has failed. Ideally, we do so in democratic, engaging way: the people whose interests are at risk are invited to voice their needs, experiences, perspectives, and concerns.

FROM CARE TO EVALUATION

Care is already present in the field of evaluation studies, despite the dominance of evaluation as a technique or method to measure practices (Dahler-Larsen, 2015; Schwandt, 2002; Simons & Greene, 2014). Evaluation theorist Thomas Schwandt, who in 1992 cited care ethics as an inspiration for evaluation, aptly rephrases Noddings's (1984) critical warning about the tendency to act as philosopher kings:

> We must keep our objective thinking tied to a relational stake at the heart of caring. When we fail to do this, we climb into clouds of abstraction, moving rapidly away from the caring situation into a domain of objective and impersonal problems where we are free to impose structure as we will. (Noddings, 1984, as cited in Schwandt, 1992, p. 141)

Thomas Schwandt reminds us of Stake's (1991) work promoting a socio-anthropological sensitivity as opposed to a scientific-technical lens for viewing human practices.

Some evaluation approaches are grounded in insights similar to those from care ethics. As mentioned, these insights regard people as interdependent and vulnerable and acknowledge the complexities of daily practices. For example, some evaluators stress the relational nature of practices (Abma & Widdershoven, 2011; Baur, Abma and Widdershoven, 2010; Abma, 2006; Visse et al., 2015). These approaches are often aimed at applying more democratic and participatory practices and regard evaluation studies as a particular pedagogy intended to create a platform for moral learning in the tradition of practical hermeneutics (Abma, Molewijk, & Widdershoven, 2008; Freeman & Hall, 2012; Freeman, Preissle, & Havick, 2010; Visse, Abma, & Widdershoven, 2012; Widdershoven, 2001; Schwandt, 2002). Examples of these approaches include democratic evaluation (Greene, 1997, 2010; Hanberger, 2016; Simons & Greene, 2014), responsive evaluation (Abma, 2008; Abma & Widdershoven, 2011; Freeman et al., 2010; Freeman & Hall, 2012; Visse et al., 2015), and transformative evaluation (Mertens, 2009). Some evaluators, like care ethicists, purposefully attend to the personal and particular features of evaluations (Abma & Stake, 2014; Kushner, 2000; Simons, 1980; Visse, Abma and Widdershoven, 2012), and some especially emphasize a caring praxis and society (Niemeijer & Visse, 2016; Visse et al., 2015; Visse & Niemeijer, 2016). They value engagement with practices and acknowledge and attend to the ambiguity in human life without finding final solutions.

These evaluation approaches share the common aim to holistically understand the evaluated program or policy from the *insider perspectives* of the participants and other stakeholders. In this holistic understanding, the evaluator pays attention to many mutually influencing factors that shape the program or policy and its context (e.g., its history, the organization and culture in which it is embedded, the persons and personalities in leadership, the political dynamics and climate, and the social interactions and relations among stakeholders). These aspects of stakeholders' relationships with one another become interwoven in the fabric of the evaluated program or policy and thus integral to program quality and effectiveness. A program or policy, therefore, should be understood as a social practice; it is never merely an intervention implemented instrumentally but always a socially, historically, politically (thus critically), and culturally determined and emerging pattern of relations, interactions, and values.

These approaches have a common awareness that evaluators should attend to the plurality of values of those whose interests or needs are at stake. It was Robert Stake (1975) who enlarged the scope of evaluation to include the issues of all possible stakeholders, based on the idea that a phenomenon has various, sometimes conflicting meanings for different stakeholders (Abma & Stake, 2001, 2014; Stake & Abma, 2005). Responsiveness to the issues of stakeholders assumes appreciation of their experiential knowledge. Methodologically, acknowledging plurality implies that the study design gradually emerges in conversation with stakeholders.

Evaluators working in these traditions are well aware of the interpretive nature of their evaluative work. The key concerns and perspectives of stakeholders are not ready-made, there to be discovered or revealed, but must be carefully received by the evaluator as a midwife. The birth of meaning is never only a matter of demonstration or representation. Human beings, including evaluators, are interpreters. To make sense of our world and endow our experiences or others' with meaning, we bring to bear our own backgrounds, training, prior experiences, desires, and standpoints. Every description is laden with interpretation. Evaluators try to stay as close to the stakeholders' accounts and narratives as possible and are skeptical about the use of conceptual frameworks in order to prevent foreclosure or reduction of data. To understand the quality of the practice, evaluators have to use their wise judgment. This type of judgment should not be understood as calculations using preordained criteria. The evaluator does not predefine a set of evaluation criteria but takes the stakeholders' issues and experiences and the evaluator's own observations as a source to assess program quality (Goodyear, Jewiss, Usinger, & Barela, 2014). Stake (1994) explains that this process is partly intuitive; one develops an understanding of program quality and later rationalizes what makes the practice good (personal communication with Abma, summer 1994; Stake & Schwandt, 2006). Schwandt (2002, 2005) refers to the Aristotelian virtue of *phronesis*, or wise judgment, to describe what it is necessary to evaluate the quality of a practice.

Wise judgment is an ordinary, empirical, quasi-aesthetic, contextual kind of knowing. Schwandt (2005) cites Berlin aptly:

> Capacity for integrating a vast amalgam of constantly changing, multicolored, evanescent, perceptually overlapping data, too many, too swift, too intermingled to be caught and pinned down and labeled like so many individual butterflies.... To seize a situation in this sense one needs to see, to be given a kind of direct, almost sensuous contact with the relevant data, and not merely to recognize their general characteristics, to classify them or reason about them, or analyze them, or reach conclusions and formulate theories about them. (Berlin, as cited in Schwandt, 2005, p. 325)

Wise judgment requires the ability to attend to the particulars of a situation, to discriminate, and to see relevant details. A wise evaluator also finds a balanced, middle-ground position between antipathy and sympathy, emotion and rationality, and does justice to and cares about all the stakeholders, or as many as possible. The Aristotelian middle-ground position is crucial in describing this practice for "the wisdom of the evaluator's findings will be little appreciated if couched in words that hurt too little or too much" (Stake, 1982, p. 80). Developing such wisdom is a never-ending process in the scholarly life of evaluator; it is fostered among novices through a developmental process which entails learning about more than methods and techniques (Visse et al., 2012). It requires a safe, friendly context that stimulates exploration and reflection on the self-as-evaluator (and on one's authority, responsibility, obligation, and so forth; see, e.g., Visse et al., 2012).

Evaluators in this tradition establish particular relationships in their evaluation as a way of challenging relationships—especially of power—in the context outside the evaluation. The purpose of evaluation is to establish equal and just relations in society and empower marginalized and precarious groups; therefore, evaluators value engagement and ownership. To effect the desired transformations, the evaluator purposefully uses the relational dimensions of evaluation and forms certain kinds of relationships—those that are accepting, respectful, and reciprocal—to promote the overall social changes desired.

Thus, the evaluator's responsibility to foster interactions among participants receives great emphasis as a way to jointly develop socially responsible practices. Active partnership, participation, and joint learning are central. In more traditional qualitative approaches, the evaluator does all the interpretive and judgmental work alone, but in an interactive approach, it is the joint responsibility of the evaluator and all the participants (including clients, patients, and citizens). In interactive evaluations, therefore, the social relations between the evaluator and various practitioners and among those practitioners are central. Interactions and relationships always matter because they shape the evaluative knowledge generated in evaluation and convey the particular norms and values the evaluation advances. It matters, for example, that evaluators kneel in the mud alongside psychiatric patients planting a garden because the relationships thus formed are respectful and accepting (Abma, 1998). With this action, the evaluators embody and live the values of respect, attentiveness, and engagement (as opposed to the more distant and hierarchical relationships in objectivist evaluation approaches). In interactive evaluations, evaluators view the social relations in the setting as more than an object of study and actively engage with the people in the setting. This broader responsibility arises from the critical consciousness and awareness that social practices are often marked by inequalities and social injustice, as well as the consequent desire to create more responsible practices through evaluative work.

Evaluators working in these traditions understand evaluation as a political practice and ask themselves *whose* interests they want to serve (Schwandt, 1997; Segerholm, 2001). They do not take social relations and societal structures for granted but critically examine and transform them. Evaluators criticize power imbalances and the status quo, often on the grounds of critical theories (Woelders & Abma, 2015). They act as social critics or commentators, opposing domination, oppression, exploitation, cruelty, and violence (Mertens, 2002; Schwandt, 2002; Segerholm, 2001). They advocate for particular silenced and marginalized groups (Lincoln, 1993), not only promoting their interests but also allowing them to participate equally in the overall learning process. The intention to pay attention to social relations, justice, and care derives from emancipatory and democratic ideals (Simons & Greene, 2014) and notions of a caring society (Tronto, 2014; Visse et al., 2015). Evaluators engage to empower people in the tradition of Paolo Freire (2007), to enhance their ability to govern their own lives, and to work toward social justice (Rosenstein, 2015) and care (Barnes, Vosman, & Conradi, 2015).

Although evaluation theory seems inclined to focus on justice and rights, we begin this book from the proposition that evaluation studies and care ethics have common interests. We assume that some evaluators are making concrete what care ethicists conceptualize and that care ethicists offer theoretical concepts that can help advance evaluation practices and theory. The specific evaluation approaches we discuss have grown as a counterpoint to approaches of evaluation that center measurement and judgment by indicators and predetermined criteria or principles and rights. The approaches discussed in this book focus on moral understanding, discursive sense-making processes, care and social justice advocacy, participation, democratization, and facilitation of diversity and pluralism.

OUTLINE OF THE BOOK

The book is divided into four parts. To aid the reader, each chapter ends with an overview of the main concepts and questions for discussion.

Part I explicitly discusses the theoretical dimensions of care and evaluation. Maurice Hamington focuses on care, competency, and knowledge in the context of a caring society. He begins with a statement on the crisis of care in current society and addresses the deficiencies in particular competences. In this Chapter 1 he argues for understanding care as a professional competency and discusses the implications for evaluation studies. Next, in Chapter 2, Karin Dahlberg focuses on the importance of understanding in care and evaluation. From a phenomenological and philosophical perspective, she explores what the process of understanding another person entails and how it contributes to a lifeworld-oriented view on evaluation. The in-betweenness of understanding, meaning of the body, concept of vulnerability, and importance of developing new epistemological approaches to understanding are raised.

Part II presents two chapters on democratic evaluation approaches. The tradition of democratic evaluation intentionally advances democratic ideals and values, notably social justice, fairness, and equity. In their Chapter 3, Helen Simons and Jennifer Greene outline the principles and values of democratic evaluation and describe how they engage with a caring ethic in their practice. They also explore crossovers, connections, and boundaries between their work and the conceptual work of some care ethicists. In Chapter 4, Anders Hanberger discusses democratic evaluation in the context of the evaluation of a Swedish program for refugee children. Hanberger connects his approach to care and aims to develop a democratic caring evaluation. He explores what a democratic caring evaluator is in relation to his concept of the practice of responsibility.

In Part III, ethics and evaluation take center stage. In her Chapter 5, "Uncontrolled Evaluation: The case of Telecare Evaluations," Jeannette Pols outlines a framework for evaluation without set criteria and argues that criteria known in advance may lead to perverse effects. She proposes an approach to evaluation inspired by empirical ethics that can be used "in the wild," or outside the laboratory conditions needed to structure evaluations.

Helen Kohlen's Chapter 6, "Evaluation for Moving Ethics in Health Care Services Towards Democratic Care: A Three Pillars Model: Education, Companionship, and Open Space," illustrates her vision of care ethics and evaluation with the example of a German project on organizational forms of ethics in health care institutions, such as Hospital Ethics Committees (HEC). Her project features an ongoing process of (self-)evaluation, foregrounds a relational perspective, and is aimed at implementing practices of democratic care.

Part IV focuses on responsive evaluation. It opens with Gustaaf Bos and Tineke Abma's Chapter 7 "Responding to Otherness: The Need for Experimental-Relational Spaces." This chapter explores the meaning of being a caring responsive evaluator in the context of care and support for people with intellectual disabilities. The chapter presents a narrative of a responsive evaluation in the field of "reversed integration" in the Netherlands. Chapter 8, "Dialogue, Difference, and Care in Responsive Enactments of a World-Becoming," by Melissa Freeman builds on the responsive evaluation of a museum-based, academically oriented program for African-American teens in the northeastern United States. She argues for a posthumanist turn in responsive evaluation based on its promises to be accountable for difference.

In Chapter 9, "Responsive Evaluation as a Way to Create Space for Sexual Diversity: A Case Example of Gay-Friendly Elderly Care," Hannah Leyerzapf, Merel Visse, Arwin de Beer, and Tineke Abma report on how responsive evaluation can open space for diversity in residential elderly care. They address LGBT older people's experiences of inclusion and participation in care settings and contribute to the development of inclusive and responsive care that structurally enhances the visibility, voice, and well-being of LGBT residents. Developing gay-friendly elderly care requires challenging exclusionary social norms. Dialogical sharing of narratives in the context of evaluation can empower LGBT older adults and stimulate understanding and shared responsibility among LGBT, heterosexual older people, and professionals.

The last chapter, Chapter 10 "Evaluation for a Caring Society: Toward New Imaginaries" is intended to provide the reader with a synthesis of the many insights, questions, and issues covered in the previous chapters. In our synthesis, we present foci for evaluators who especially aim to nurture a caring society. If our foci break new ground, they provide new conceptions of the fundamentals and practice of evaluation.

REFERENCES

Abma, T. A., & Stake, R. (2014). Science of the particular. An advocacy for naturalistic case study in health. *Qualitative Health* Research, *24*(8), 1150–1161. doi:10.1177/1049732314543196

Abma, T. A., & Widdershoven, G. A. M. (2011). Evaluation as a relationally responsive practice. In N. Denzin & Y. S. Lincoln (Eds.). *Qualitative research. Sage handbook* (pp. 669–680). Los Angeles, CA: SAGE.

Abma, T., & Widdershoven, G. (2008). Evaluation as social relation. *Evaluation, 14*(2), 209–225.

Abma, T. (2006). The practice and politics of responsive evaluation. *American Journal of Evaluation, 27*(1), 31–43.

Abma, T. A. (1998). Storytelling as inquiry in a mental hospital. *Qualitative Health Research, 8*(6), 821–838.

Barnes, M. Knops, A., Newman, J., & Sullivan, H. (2004). Recent research. The micro-politics of deliberation: Case studies in public participation. *Contemporary Politics, 10*(2), 93–110.

Baur, V. E., Van Elteren, A. H. G., Nierse, C. J., & Abma, T. A. (2010). Dealing with distrust and power dynamics: Asymmetric relations among stakeholders in responsive evaluation. *Evaluation, 16*(3), 233–248.

Baur, V., Abma, T. A., & Widdershoven, G. A. M. (2010). Participation of older people in evaluation: Mission impossible? *Evaluation and Program Planning, 33*(3), 238–45.

Dahler-Larsen, P. (2015). The evaluation society: Critique, contestability and skepticism. *Spazio Filosofico, 1*(13), *21–36.*

Engster, D. (2007). *The heart of justice. Care ethics and political theory.* Oxford, England: Oxford University Press.

Fisher, B., & Tronto, J. (1990). Toward a feminist theory of caring. In E. Abel & M. Nelson (Eds.), *Circles of care* (pp. 36–54), Albany: State University of New York Press.

Freeman, M., & Hall, J .N. (2012). Responsive evaluation of a professional development school partnership. *American Journal of Evaluation, 33,* 483-495. doi:10.1177/1098214012443728

Freeman, M., Preissle, J., & Havick, S. (2010). Moral knowledge and responsibilities *New Directions for Evaluation* (pp. 45–57).

Freire, P. (2007). *Pedagogy of the oppressed.* New York, NY: Continuum.

Gilligan, C. (1982). *In a Different Voice.* Boston, MA: Harvard University Press.

Goodyear, L., Jewiss, Usinger, J., & Barele, E. (Eds.). (2014). *Qualitative inquiry in evaluation,* San Francisco, CA: Jossey-Bass.

Greene, J. C. (1997). Evaluation as advocacy. *American Journal of Evaluation, 18,* 25–35.

Greene, J. C. (2010). Serving the public good. *Evaluation and Program Planning, 33*(2), 197–200.

Hanberger, A. (2016). The role of evaluation in local school governance in Sweden: Editorial introduction. *Education Inquiry,* 7(3), 211–216.

Held, V. (2015). Care and Justice, still. In: Engster, D., Hamington, M. *Care Ethics & Political Theory.* Oxford, England: Oxford University Press.

Kushner, S. (2000). *Personalizing evaluation.* London, England: SAGE.

Laugier, S. (2014). Care: Ethics as a politic of the ordinary. Talk at the Seminar Series on Care: Care practices towards a recasting of ethics. Oxford Martin School, Oxford, England. Retrieved from https://www.youtube.com/watch?v=THHwB0pXmFk&list=UUmXB98lpzelFrlryV2llXUQ

Leget, C., van Nistelrooij, I., & Visse, M. (2017). Beyond demarcation: Care ethics as an interdisciplinary field of inquiry. *Nursing Ethics.* 0969733017707008

Lincoln, Y. S. (1993). I and thou: Method, voice, and roles in research with the silenced. In D. McLaughlin & W. Tierney (Eds.), *Naming silenced lives* (pp. 29–47), New York, NY: Routledge.

Mertens, D. M. (2009). *Transformative research and evaluation.* New York, NY: Guilford.

Niemeijer, A., & Visse, M. A. (2016). Challenging standard concepts of 'humane' care through relational auto-ethnography. *Inclusion, 4*(4), 168–175.

Noddings, N. (1984). *Caring: A feminine approach to ethics and moral education.* Berkeley, CA: University of California Press.

Rosenstein, B., Desivilya Syna, H. (2015). *Evaluation and social justice in complex socio-political contexts.* New Directions for Evaluation, 146.

Sayer, A. (2011). *Why things matter to people. Social science, values and ethical life.* New York, NY: Cambridge University Press.

Schwandt, T. A. (1992). Better living through evaluation? Images of progress shaping evaluation practice. *Evaluation Practice, 13*(2), 135–144.

Schwandt, T. A. (1997). Whose interests are being served? Program evaluation as conceptual practice of power. In L. Mabry (Ed.), *Evaluation and the post-modern dilemma. Advances in Program Evaluation* (Vol. 3, pp. 89–104). Greenwich, CT: JAI Press.

Schwandt, T. A. (2002). *Evaluation practice reconsidered.* New York, NY: Peter Lang.

Schwandt, T. S. (2005). On modeling our understanding of the practice fields. *Pedagogy, Culture and Society, 13*(3), 313–332.

Segerholm, C. (2001). Evaluation as responsibility, conscience, and conviction. In K. E. Ryan & T. S. Schwandt (Eds.), *Exploring evaluator role and identity* (pp. 87–102). Greenwich, CT: Information Age.

Simons, H. (1980). *Towards a science of the singular.* Norwich, England: University of East Anglia.

Simons, H., & Greene, J. C. (2014, October). *Against the odds but worth it: The value of democratic evaluation in contemporary society.* Keynote address at the European Evaluation Society, Dublin, Ireland.

Solnit, R. (2017). *The mother of all questions.* Chicago, IL: Haymarket Books.

Stake, R. E. (1975). To evaluate an arts program. In R. E. Stake (Ed.), *Evaluating the arts in education: A responsive approach* (pp. 13–31). Columbus, OH: Merrill.

Stake, R. E. (1982, August). How sharp should the evaluator's teeth be? *Evaluation News,* pp. 79–80.

Stake, R. E. (1991). Retrospective on "the countenance of educational evaluation." In M. W. McLaughlin & D. C. Phillips (Eds.), *Evaluation and education: At quarter century, ninetieth yearbook of the National Society for the Study of Education (NSSE)* (pp. 67–88). Chicago, IL: University of Chicago Press.

Stake, R. E., & Abma, T. A. (2005). Responsive evaluation. In S. Matheson (Ed.), *Encyclopedia of evaluation* (pp. 376–379). Thousand Oaks, CA: SAGE.

Stake, R. E., & Schwandt, T. S. (2006). On discerning quality in evaluation. In I. F. Shaw, J. C. Greene, & M. M. Mark (Eds.), *The SAGE handbook of evaluation* (pp. 404–418). London, England: SAGE.

Tronto, J.C. (1993). *Moral boundaries: A political argument for an ethic of care.* New York, NY: Routledge.

Tronto, J. C. (2013). *Caring democracy: Markets, equality and justice.* New York, NY: New York University Press.

Tronto, J. C. (2014). Moral boundaries after twenty years: From limits to possibilities. Ethics of care: Present and new directions. In G. Olthuis, H. Kohlen, & H. Heier (Eds.). *Moral boundaries redrawn: The significance of Joan Tronto's Argument for political theory, professional ethics and care as practice. Ethics of care* (Vol. 3, pp. 9–29, 215–229). Leuven, Belgium: Peeters.

Van Nistelrooij, I. (2014). *Sacrifice. A care ethical reappraisal of sacrifice and self-sacrifice.* (PhD dissertation Utrecht, University of Humanistic Studies).

Visse, M. A., Abma, T. A., & Widdershoven, G. A. M. (2012). Relational responsibilities in responsive evaluation. *Evaluation and Program Planning, 35,* 97–104.

Visse, M. A., Abma, T. A., & Widdershoven, G. A. M. (2015). Practising political *Welfare, 9*(2), 164–182.

Visse, M., & Niemeijer, A. (2016). Autoethnography as a praxis of care: The *International Journal of Qualitative Inquiry, 16*(3), 301–312.

Widdershoven, G. A. M., & Huijer, M. (2001). The fragility of care. An encounter between Nussbaum's Aristotelean ethics and ethics of care. *International Journal in Philosophy and Theology, 62,* 304–316.

Woelders, S., & Abma, T. (2015). A different light on normalization: Critical theory and responsive evaluation studying social justice in participation practices. *New Directions for Evaluation, 146*, 9–18. doi:10.1002/ev.20116

THE PHOTO-STORY OF THE CAREFREESTATE

Janine Schrijver
Introduced by Tineke Abma and Merel Visse

The images of this special volume were taken in the central kitchen of the "Carefreestate" in a large city of the Netherlands by Dutch photographer Janine Schrijver. We greatly appreciate her generous gesture to include them in this volume.

In the city of Rotterdam in the Netherlands, a new initiative, run by and for citizens is called the *Carefreestate* (De zorgvrijstaat). Ironically, this community-inspired initiative is all about caring for each other. It is not carefree, but care work done by people from and for the local neighborhood, freed from state control and professional expertise. It ranges from preparing and cooking meals, to sharing a dinner together. From doing groceries for older people who are unable to go outside anymore, to supporting other neighbors with their tax forms. It is an example of a bottom-up, nongovernmental, strong social infrastructure that puts 'care' at its center. Care and care work are not tangible. But the marginal social product of care is great. Care gives numerous contributions to human and social capital.

Evaluation for a Caring Society, pages 17–20

Like the title of this initiative the photos also show an ambivalence. The political context during which these photographs were taken, was characterized by Dutch welfare retrenchments due to the financial crisis, enforcement of the Social Support Act and decentralization of welfare services from the national government to local municipalities by promoting informal care. These policy measures were combined with a discourse of participation society, active citizenship, neighborhood power, and empowerment. The Carefreestate was a citizen initiative as a response to cutbacks in professional care and welfare. An initiative run by and for the neighborhood. The photos make us wonder: who are these women, cooking? Are they voluntarily doing this work, or are they expected—based on social norms and roles—to carry out this care work? The photos invite us to ponder upon the idea of transferring care work from welfare and health care professionals to citizens. From a care ethical perspective we may critically interrogate if the Dutch policy is not reinforcing the 'moral boundary' between the private and public domain; that is to say, confining care work to the private domain, something carried out by women, without their democratic involvement in allocating care? As Joan Tronto (1993) reminds us: moral boundaries are reinforcing hierarchies in societies.

On a global level, the United Nations Program on Sustainable Development proposes an Agenda that explicitly addresses care work and the importance of gender equality. The woman who cooks, named Zaitone Osman, has a migrant background. One can see she is proud. We also see other women with a migrant background helping her out. Is this a daughter, a girlfriend? Why don't we see White women? Or White men? Are they paid or unpaid care workers? Evaluating this Carefreestate initiative from a care ethical perspective leads us to the question whether it reproduces or sets up new hierarchies, for example between those who coordinate care (in this case, paid, White Dutch professionals) and those who are doing the care work (indeed unpaid female, minority, volunteers). This distinction between "taking care of" and "caring for," both crucial phases in the process of care (Tronto, 1993), reproduces power positions between groups in society, and it devalues care work. That is to say, the caring labor is passed on in society to those with the least social status. Symbolically, this leads to a devaluation of care work. Another asymmetry that requires investigation is the assignment of care work among neighbors; why are certain neighbors acting as volunteers, and others not? Are we looking at the reality of what Joan Tronto so aptly calls *privileged irresponsibility* (Tronto 1993)? This denotes a situation where those in a privileged position are able not to take responsibility for care. First of all, they have the financial resources to take care of themselves. Secondly, they are in the position not to attend to the care for others; they do not have to do caring work themselves. Caring work, then, is something done by "others" (pp. 146–147).

This concerning development, the care work that is done by a small portion of society, is worsened by other trends like outsourcing, offshoring, and the privatization of care work. All these threaten the equal division of care work. Collective identities and interests based on gender, race, and income level shape our institutions and economic inequality. We see a revolutionary fist that reminds us of Che Guevarra. The clenched fist has internationally become the symbol of labor protest, the upraised arm is as Sarah Ahmed (2017) recognizes "a revolutionary limb; a promise of what is to come" (p. 85). Yet, we wonder who chose this symbol. Whose revolution is this? Was it chosen by the women? Is the voluntary work a way to participate, get out of their houses, a way to a paid job? Freedom, even? Is it a gateway to more social contact or a paid job in the neighborhood? We know such expectations hardly get rewarded in the Netherlands (Slootjes, 2017). Dutch migrant integration policies assume that paid work is the ticket to integration. Lately, more pressure is put on ethnic minority women and punitive measures are used to find work, but possibilities for such employment on the side of employers are not created. Finding a paid job is primarily an individual responsibility, and as this is hard due to discrimination on the labor market, the policy focus on paid work is disempowering. It makes us wonder at what price this care work is done. Who takes, for instance, care of the children and family? And, if nobody does, the volunteering work just adds up to all other care work that needs to be done, which raises the question how women balance all those activities. At the cost of their own health perhaps?

These women work in a kitchen. We see the circumstances. For Dutch standards very plain. No extras, no luxury. A damp room. One of the pots on the fire is missing a handle. One could easily burden oneself when picking up the hot pan. Not too safe... Why was this not repaired? What does this say about the value endowed to the care work? What does it say about the social status and symbolic power of minority women?

The photos raised many questions and concerns, but above all it triggered our curiosity into the lived experiences and voice of the woman so prominently facing us. What was her story? How did she feel about the voluntary work? What kind of future did she envision for her children, her daughters perhaps? Therefore, Tineke took the initiative to meet and talk with her. On a late afternoon in the end of December 2017 Tineke met with Zaitone Osman. She welcomed Tineke in her kitchen and spoke about her childhood in Irak, how she fled from the war to Iran with her parents and later with her husband and children through Syria to The Netherlands. Zaitone shared her experiences on her precarious position in Dutch society, her dreams and impressive work with and for women. The conversation formed the basis of a poem entitled 'I am Zaitone.' Tineke crafted the poem using the words and language of Zaitone, translated it into English, and checked with Zaitone whether she recognized it, which she indeed did.

REFERENCES

Ahmed, S. (2017). *Living a feminist life.* Durham, NC: Duke University Press.

Slootjes, J. (2017). *Narratives of meaningful endurance: The role of sense of coherence in health and employment of ethnic minority women.* Porefschriftenprinten, Ede. PhD Thesis, VU University Amsterdam.

Tronto, J.C. (1993). *Moral boundaries. A political argument for an ethic of care,* New York, NY: Routledge.

I am Zaitone
By Tineke Abma, in collaboration with Zaitone Osman

I am Zaitone
I am a mother of four
I was born in Irak

(On her youth)
I was just a little girl
When Saddam came I was eight years old
I heard the bombings all the time
That's what I remember
The sound of breaking glass, that's what I remember
I had to obey the teachers
I was forced
I cannot belief
saying I had to, otherwise my father…
I am Kurdish
I learned Arabic
With my parents I fled
Ten days I walked, it was cold
In an Iranian camp I survived

(On her becoming)
I was trained and I worked
When I came here I went to school again
I learned Dutch
Still I am a minority
But with my Dutch I can connect
I connect with all the women
I drink coffee with the mothers
I know more over than hundred women
Let's start reading to our children, I said
I proposed
I initiated
That is how I started
I went to a Talk Show in the library
That is where I met
I forgot her name
I think perhaps Irene?
I accepted her help with writing letters

(On women)
I want to support women
That's what I love to do
I see many work so hard inside their homes
Their strength isn't always acknowledged, I regret
So I listen
I really listen, opening my heart
And I am patient
Listening and being patient, I feel
That's important, I think
I understand
Their hardship, I sense, and their stress
They say I can sense everything
I cannot solve their problems
But I can be there, showing them the way

(On the fist)
I don't like the fist
The fist is of men, I grief
Over male aggression, I grief
I value women's ways
I value using our brains and our hearts
I value education

(On religion)
I am deeply religious
I was struck and wear a scarf since
Not because I am obliged to
Not because I have to
I do not belief in external force
Sometimes I see girls in the tram
putting their scarfs away, and I feel sorry
I belief, it comes from inside

(On being a volunteer)
Four days a week I work
I coordinate
I organize
I cook
I buy food at the street market
The spacy kitchen, I like
And I like women around
I open the window, so the smell gets out
people come and taste, I offer food

I share
I share a healthy meal
I do not get paid
But I dream
A social worker I would like to be
I try
I have no diploma
I am too old?
My girls, they push me, I am eager
I consider going back to school
I am curious
I want them to be proud of me
I want to be a role model
I am an example
I am Zaitone

PART I

THEORETICAL REFLECTIONS ON A CARING SOCIETY

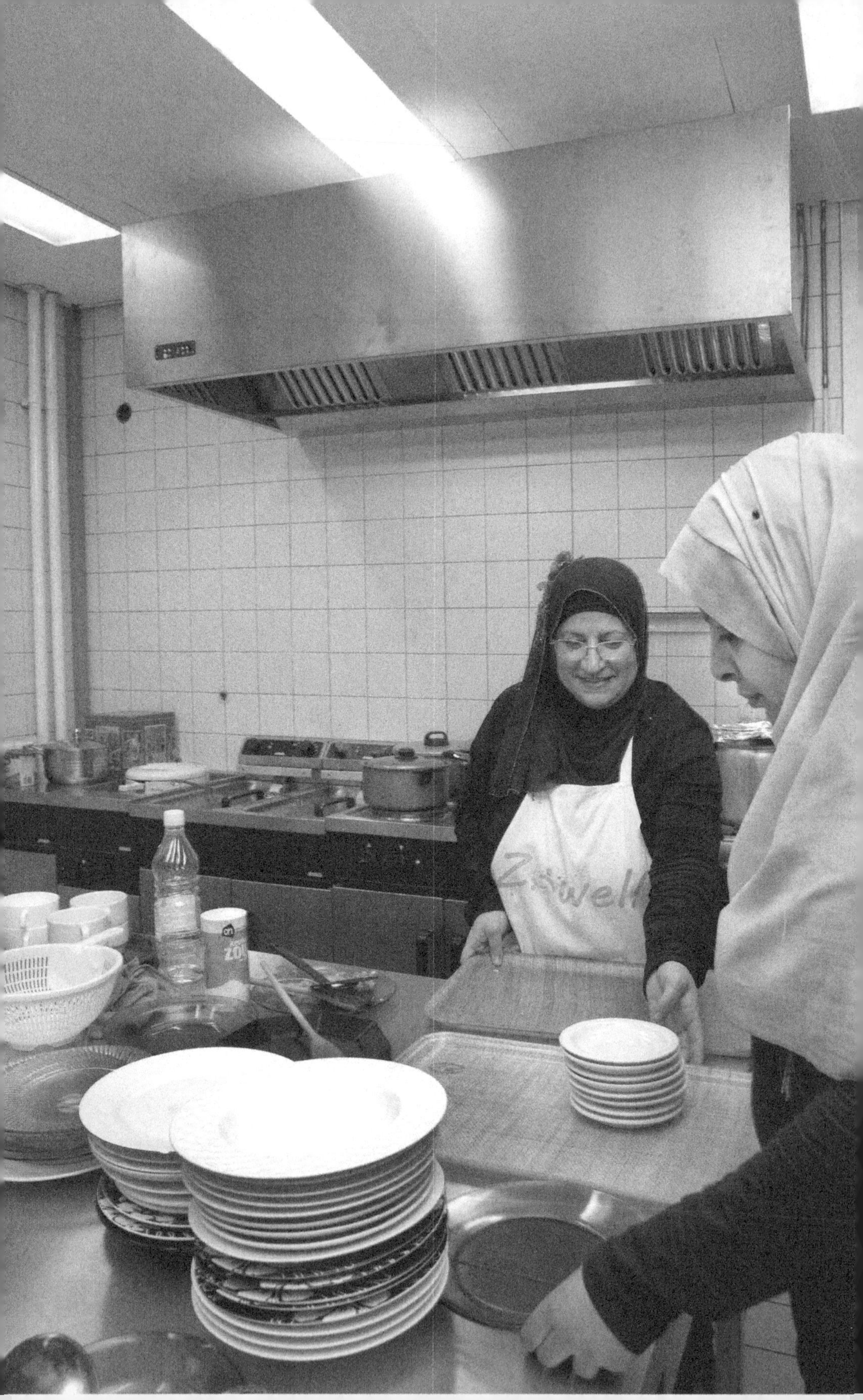

CHAPTER 1

CARE, COMPETENCY, AND KNOWLEDGE

Maurice Hamington
Portland State University

Many authors have lamented the contemporary existence of a social "crisis of care." This crisis manifests itself differently depending upon the context. Author Madeleine Bunting (2016) declared on a recent BBC broadcast:

> Social care is in crisis; news stories almost every day report on the growing care deficit for the ageing population and for adults with long term health conditions and disabilities. Nothing illustrates more starkly the systematic undervaluing of care in our culture. This is the labor of caring for those who need help with daily life: getting up, dressing, feeding themselves, washing and keeping their homes clean.

Bunting (2016) refers to a crisis of care delivery systems and caring labor. Crises of care have been variously declared in healthcare (Benner & Philips), in migration practice and policy (Benería, 2004), in education (Noddings, 1988), and in economic practices (Engster, 2007), to name a few examples. In each case, there is a perceived lack of human connection,

Evaluation for a Caring Society, pages 27–48

nurturing, or meeting needs in times of vulnerability. Despite the general Western idealization of autonomy and independence, all humans are vulnerable beings who require significant care at various times in their lives to both survive and flourish. Claiming a "crisis" is a means for calling attention to an under-attended deficit of modernity. Yet, this crisis is not simply the lack of the existence of care or systems for delivering it, but can be also described as a deficiency of competent care. Without adequate competency, many actions delivered under the guise of care can be experienced as cold, indifferent, incomplete, perfunctory, bureaucratic, and generally unconcerned with the one cared for. Authentic care demands skilled responsiveness to the individual. What is suggested in this chapter is that competency is not simply a technical professionalism but also entails emotional intelligence, responsiveness, and inquiry—all elements of care. An expansive definition of the knowledge that supports professionalism is required in the face of a widespread crisis of deficient care. Understanding care as a professional competency also indicates a need for evaluation.

Participating in the recognition of a contemporary crisis of care is the attention of late devoted to care ethics as having both moral and practical significance. Care ethics describes an approach to moral action that is challenging and laborious. Unable to fall back on formulaic ethical rubrics to answer questions of right action, authentic deep care requires time, effort, risk, and emotional investment to locate the emergent normative action for a particular person in a specific context. In other words, caring must be responsive. This chapter suggests an additional burden for the one caring by arguing that there is an epistemic demand to effective and responsive care. Robust care requires the one caring to be an active inquirer and a lifelong learner committed to knowledge both broadly and specifically construed. This epistemic demand is true for both individuals involved in ordinary daily caring as well as those who engage in caring professions and policy makers.

After offering a definition of a performative and political care ethics, this chapter suggests a two-source knowledge structure that includes both concrete and generalized knowledge as a prerequisite for care. Although concrete knowledge—the particular, local knowledge of the one cared for—dominates the care literature, generalized knowledge—skills and information that can be used across different individuals—is the most commonly referenced attribute of the competent professional. However, in this chapter I claim that both generalized and concrete knowledge are essential to competent care. Bringing this two-part epistemic lens to care ethics reframes caring away from the exclusive considerations of what occurs within dyadic relationships to include reliable social evidence thus introducing a significant third party to the experience of quality care. In other words, the one caring is not just responsive to the particular one cared for but must also engage social and scientific understanding of what it means to care.

The two-source claim for care knowledge has implications for all forms of effective care, but this chapter pays particular attention to the delivery and assessment of professionals. Given the two-source theory of caring knowledge, the discussion then turns to assessing care along concrete and generalized dimensions.

CARE ETHICS

The term *care ethics* entered the lexicon of Western philosophy in the 1980's as an alternative approach to morality. Emphasizing relationships, care ethics valorizes context and emotion in a richer manner than traditional philosophical approaches. Over the decades since the introduction of the term, various theorists have expanded and enriched the understanding of care. Care ethics' most prolific contributor, Nel Noddings, has emphasized the attentive and responsive aspects of care (1984, 2002, 2010). Eva Kittay's (Kittay, 2015; Kittay & Feder, 2003) work has explored the role of disability and vulnerability in caring relationships. Michael Slote (2007, 2010) has contributed a richer understanding of the centrality of empathy and sentiment in caring actions. Joan Tronto (1993, 2013), Selma Sevenhuijsen (1998), Fiona Robinson (1999, 2011), Virginia Held (2006), and Dan Engster (2007, 2015) have helped make care ethics a significant approach to political theorizing. Increasingly, scholars have found care ethics an attractive way to understand the interrelated and interdependent nature of human existence, highlighting new aspects of care as well as new applications.

Although notoriously difficult to define, the most common characterization of care ethics is as a relational approach to morality. For example, Carol Gilligan (2011) defines care as:

> An ethic grounded in voice and relationships, in the importance of everyone having a voice, being listened to carefully (in their own right and on their own terms) and heard with respect. An ethics of care directs our attention to the need for responsiveness in relationships (paying attention, listening, responding) and to the costs of losing connection with oneself or with others. Its logic is inductive, contextual, psychological, rather than deductive or mathematical. (online interview)

Gilligan's (2011) definition correctly emphasizes the relational, but for this project I draw attention to care's epistemic aspects, which, for example, are embedded but not explicated in Gilligan's (2011) emphasis on responsiveness above.

I have previously employed an understanding of care that names its physicality and highlights its epistemic implications:

> Care is a political embodied performance, every iteration of which has the potential to contribute to our dynamic sense of moral identity, adds to our disruptive knowledge of the other, and supports the notion that ethical understanding is a mind–body activity that is ripe for autopoetic development. (Hamington 2015, p. 279)

This definition attempts to fit the complexity of care into a single sentence. Let me explain this definition a bit as it underlies what follows in this chapter. First, by claiming that care is a performance, I am noting that care is ultimately an action in the world that is witnessed by others and at the very least witnessed by myself. The performativity of care is an important lens for understanding how it can be enacted in more or less competent ways, which is in turn essential for assessing care. The body is always involved in the delivery and receiving of care, although its role is often overlooked (Hamington, 2004). Because the body's caring actions involve others and is witnessed by others, caring activity has power and political implications. Although moral philosophy has a tendency to focus on adjudicating individual acts in isolation (i.e., "What is the right thing to do?"), caring actions have a habitual structure that can be mapped onto any number of new situations. The repetition of caring actions influences our identity in terms of the extent to which we understand ourselves to be caring persons, but more importantly the iterations of care means that we can reflect on our actions and improve them. Care is a moral ideal (Noddings, 1984), not in a fixed and unobtainable utopian sense but rather it is a moral ideal that we can engage with on a daily basis. Knowledge of the other is crucial for care. That knowledge can be disruptive and pull us out of our self concerns to make us other directed. Sometimes that knowledge encroaches upon us in seemingly innocuous ways as when someone who is in distress approaches us. Other times we can actively pursue knowledge that informs caring. It is the vigorous pursuit of knowledge in animating care that is emphasized in this chapter. Taken altogether, the performative definition of care describes relational embodied beings who operate like dynamic systems, adapting and connecting through learning and caring.

As hinted at in the beginning of this article, we often speak of care as if it is a binary: either care is given or it is not. However the contemporary crisis of care is not just about a complete lack of care but also about incomplete or incompetent care. For the purpose of establishing an enlarged notion of competency, we presume that the experience of care exists on a continuum: Care has a range of depth and quality. Tronto (1993) offers a claim about the significance of action over disposition that hints at something more than a binary understanding of care: "Intending to provide care, even accepting responsibility for it, but then failing to provide good care, means that in the end the need for care is not met" (p. 133). Care is generally offered and received on a continuum of effectiveness rather than a dichotomous care/

not care experience. Tronto's (1993) reference to providing "good" care is of particular interest to this project. What is involved in providing good care? What constitutes providing professional care? An important response to these questions regarding the range of quality care is knowledge.

KNOWLEDGE AS A PREREQUISITE FOR CARE

Although not always articulated, we intuitively know that caring and knowing are intimately linked. On the one hand, I simply cannot care about anything that I do not know about. On the other hand, familiarity creates the opportunity for care. Time, presence, and proximity spent with another individual have the potential to foster connection, empathy, and ultimately caring actions.

The idea that knowledge is a prerequisite for care is present among care theorists even when epistemic claims are implicit rather than explicitly identified, as in Gilligan's (2011) definition above. This implicit presence of knowledge production can be witnessed in the discussions of care and empathy. A number of care theorists have identified the significant role of empathy in igniting care (Verducci 2000; Noddings 2002; Slote 2007, 2010; Pulcini 2016), even if empathy is not a sufficient condition of care (Pulcini 2016, p. 7; Hamington, 2016). Empathy requires knowledge, whether it is cognitive empathy (perspective taking) or emotive empathy (feeling with). One has to know something of the other to have mental or visceral empathy for them. Empathy is a knowledge driven state even if it is not frequently characterized in that manner. The general point is that caring, like empathy, requires knowledge. Accordingly, that which I superficially know, I can only care about superficially. You might respond that when disaster strikes halfway around the world, we care about what happens to the unfamiliar people affected, and you would be correct. However, in identifying the object of care as fellow human beings, my inherent knowledge has grown exponentially. Shared humanity, by implication indicates shared embodiment and all that it entails, which drives my level of understanding higher even if I don't know the victims specifically. If I further learn about the particular lives and stories of the disaster victims, the potential for my caring increases.

Care and knowledge are intertwined. The more I care about someone or something, the more I am motivated to learn about them. When we meet someone who we enjoy being around, the tendency is to inquire into that person's life and circumstances. Caring motivates inquiry. It is difficult to imagine someone who deeply cares for another person without having or desiring significant knowledge about that individual. Expanding the circle of those cared for requires knowledge. Because of the prominent role that knowledge plays in caring, I claim that competent responsive care is a form of inquiry and entails an epistemic burden. Several theorists have addressed care's epistemological dimension.

Vrinda Dalmiya (2002) describes care as a knowledge saturated skill (p. 50). For Dalmiya care is a reliable knowledge source describing a form of inquiry. She describes, "Caring as an adjective of the knower is relevant for all knowledge because it signals an effort necessary for both knowledge of things and of selves" (p. 47). Similarly, Lorraine Code (2015) contends that care is a vital and undervalued aspect of all epistemic endeavors including scientific inquiry. Challenging the legacy of positivist science and dominant forms of disengaged objectivity, Code suggests that the notion of the impartial detached researcher is a fiction.

The entrenched image of the dispassionate, disconnected knower works with a curiously implausible conception of subjectivity: a person detached from the world who does not care in the slightest about what he or she knows, whose affectivity is excised from her or his intellectual life, and who need not—borrowing Karen Barad's (2007) apt phrase—evince any concern about "meeting the universe halfway." How, one must ask, could such a person be or be imagined, other than between the covers of an orthodox Anglo-American epistemology text? (Code, 2015).

Despite a philosophical tradition that distances emotion from epistemology, Code (2015) and others suggest not only that the dichotomy is false but also that there is efficacy in the combination. Code's observation is particularly useful as we consider the caring professional. Dispassionate detachment is sometimes associated with professionalism. Dalmiya, Code, and others are attempting to diminish this association. Extending their work, I claim that care is an element in all forms of professionalism given that no one is in an isolated profession segregated from interaction with others.

Recasting care as knowledge based and understood as a form of inquiry points to elements that can be used to assess the competence of caregivers. Next, an analysis of two broad knowledge categories necessary for good care is explored.

TWO-SOURCE MODEL FOR CARING KNOWLEDGE: THE GENERALIZED AND THE CONCRETE

Early in the development of care ethics, Seyla Benhabib (1987) authored a significant article critiquing traditional moral and political theories as emphasizing the perspective of a generalized and interchangeable subject over the particular circumstances of specific individuals. According to Benhabib (1987), traditional morality as governed by justice and rights requires framing everyone as the same and treating them as equals. Benhabib favors care ethics as foregrounding the significance of understanding a specific individual or "concrete other":

> The standpoint of the concrete other... requires us to view each and every rational being as an individual with a concrete history, identity, and affective-emotional constitution. In assuming this standpoint, we abstract from what constitutes our commonality, and focus on individuality. (p. 159)

To describe two categories that make up the knowledge necessary for effective care, I adapt Benhabib's use of the terms *generalized* and *concrete.* Although her project addressed perspective taking and understanding the constructed "self" of moral theory, I am using these terms to describe epistemic categories necessary for care. Specifically, concrete knowledge is my designation for local, contextual knowledge that largely comes from the one cared for. Generalized knowledge is understanding of the habits and skills necessary to deliver care. Both forms of knowledge are necessary for competent care. Mapping these categories onto health care, for example, both concrete knowledge of a particular patient and the generalized knowledge of best medical care practices are needed for effective care.

Concrete Local Knowledge

"Concrete knowledge" as it is used here defines the responsive local knowledge that derives from the one cared for. If care is to be understood as responsive, concrete local knowledge is crucial. The existing philosophical literature on care ethics emphasizes concrete knowledge by stressing terms such as *engrossment, attentiveness,* and *presence.* In Noddings' (1984) early work, she used the word engrossment (p. 17) to describe the kind of focus the one caring needed to have on the one cared for: "an open, nonselective receptivity to the cared-for" (Noddings, 2005, p. 15). Concerned about misunderstanding that engrossment implied the kind of regard offered by a lover, Noddings (2010) began referring to care as requiring receptive attention (p. 47). "Attention" is the term most often used to describe the means of acquiring the concrete local knowledge necessary for care. For example, Tronto (1993, 2013) describes attentiveness and responsibility as the central values of care (p. 127, p. 34). Sevenhuijsen (1998) frames the epistemological challenge of attentiveness that maintains the autonomy and dignity of the one-cared for: "The recipient of care is, for her, not an 'object to be known', but someone to whom she listens, whom she tries to understand, and with whom she communicates" (p. 61). In one sense, attention is a means to an end because attention brings forth specific concrete knowledge of the one cared for. However, as Sevenhuijsen's claim points out, ultimately attention describes *both* means and ends. The acts of listening, questioning, and seeking to understand are indeed caring and are experienced as caring by the one-cared for. However, the process also results in concrete particular information that has the potential to further improve the efficacy of care. Means and ends are intermingled in the competent practices of care.

Developing concrete knowledge of another person usually requires time and attention. Concrete knowledge can consist of *propositional knowledge* exemplified in statements such as "Mary is a diabetic," "Mary has four children," and/or "Mary is upset about a recent break up with a partner." The more time and attention spent with an individual, the more propositional knowledge that can be gleaned. However, concrete knowledge can be complemented by tacit knowledge. As Michael Polanyi (1966) famously states, "we can know more than we can tell" (p. 4). Tacit knowledge is captured in the subtle and nuanced capacities of our senses, which are often beyond words. Much of this tacit knowledge is visceral and felt, and yet it is useful in fleshing out concrete propositional knowledge by facilitating understanding of the whole person who is the one cared for. As Hans Reinders (2010) describes, caregivers who are able to obtain tacit knowledge "are able to see and understand the emotions, state of minds, behaviors, body languages of these clients in ways that cannot be separated from these relationships" (p. 36).

Andries Baart's theory of presence offers an approach to obtaining concrete local knowledge that manifests the intermingling of means (attentiveness) and ends (concrete knowledge) creating a rich opportunity to obtain tacit knowledge by setting aside the common professional desire to immediately problem solve and instead advocates being present to the one care for. "Problem solving can indeed emerge from their efforts, but that is not their overt intention nor is problem solving the criterion of success" (Baart & Vosman, 2011, p. 185). Baart (2002) describes a theory of professional care that requires time. "Presence practitioners have time and take time, and they work to ensure that the time available remains 'free' (i.e., not filled with secret plans and professional intentions)" (p. 4). Time spent with someone transforms the unfamiliar to the familiar and builds trust. Presence also tacitly communicates the importance and dignity of the one cared for, allowing them to gain their voice and setting the stage for their active participating in the caring relationship. According to Klaver and Baart (2011), the presence practitioner's "first and foremost aim is to learn to know the other in a meaningful relationship, through which he or she will come to dignity" (p. 687). Note the epistemic language in the previous sentence: "know the other." Of course, time is a very precious commodity in healthcare today, hence the aforementioned crisis of care. Market and resource concerns place ever increasing pressure on medical professionals to spend as little time as possible with patients in the name of efficiency making presence a particularly difficult challenge. In this environment, the time necessary for acquiring concrete local knowledge of the one cared for creates a tension in resisting shorter patient exposure.

Baart's theory of presence implicitly addresses the challenge of power differential in caring relationships (Klaver, Elst, & Baart, 2014, p. 760). Professionals desiring to care often have to overcome the alienation that comes with their position of power in society. Although presence does not negate social power imbalance, it mitigates some of the challenges of information flow when the one cared for does not occupy the same perceived social status as the caregiver. Presence breeds familiarity and connection that disrupts perceived social distance including those invested with power. In regard to caring practices, power and privilege can be a barrier to a caring relationship that supports understanding the particulars and context of the one cared for.

In addition to the proximal and temporal structure of presence in generating the local knowledge needed for effective care, there are the skills necessary for active inquiry. María Puig de la Bellacasa (2011) addresses the epistemological implications of care: "Adequate care requires knowledge and curiosity regarding the needs of an 'other'" (p. 98). Puig de la Bellacasa (2012) proposes "thinking with care" (p. 198) as a political approach to creating healthy community and common cause with unfamiliar others. For Puig de la Bellacasa (2011), the particularism of care demands inquiry. Everything and everybody comes with a context, and to truly make a connection and understand them, takes labor. However, Puig de la Bellacasa (2012) warns that caring does not mean idealized harmonious relationships. Authentic caring entails understanding and respecting difference and disagreement: "Thinking with care is a response led by awareness of the efforts it takes to cultivate relatedness in collective and accountable knowledge construction without negating dissent" (p. 205). Puig de la Bellacasa (2012) suggests that caring represents a twofold epistemic challenge. First, to care is to recognize that every person comes with a complex set of circumstances, therefore requiring the time and energy to care with any depth. The second challenge is to care even when the other is disagreeable. Caring only for those for whom one is in accord is another form of superficiality. Given Puig de la Bellacasa's observations, the skills of responsive inquiry are actually a generalized form of knowledge that belongs in the next discussion on generalized knowledge but the fruits of these skills contribute to concrete knowledge.

Care as inquiry is dictated by its fundamental character of responsiveness. The problem of existing as discrete beings is that we can never fully know others—We cannot inhabit their bodies and brains. Nevertheless, human beings have the perceptual capacity to attend to and learn a great deal about individual others, therefore narrowing the chasm between the one and the many. The acquisition of concrete knowledge is important for the information it elicits and, as Sevenhuijsen (1998), Baart (2002), and Puig de la Bellacasa (2012) each point out, the effort at gaining concrete knowledge also expresses a caring character that benefits the one caring and the one cared for.

Generalized Knowledge

As mentioned above, much of the existing literature on care ethics supports the necessity of local specific knowledge as a prerequisite to responsive caring by describing the importance of empathy and attention. The emphasis among care theorists on concrete knowledge is in part a reaction to the scientific, political, and social valorization of generalized knowledge but it does not negate the significance of such knowledge. In addition, the weight placed on concrete knowledge stems from a definition of care that concentrates on the relationship of the one caring and the one cared for. Noddings' (2005) definition is exemplary: "A *caring relation* is, in its most basic form, a connection or encounter between two human beings—a carer and a recipient of care, or cared-for" (p. 15). Furthermore, Noddings indicates that caring involves meeting the "expressed needs" of an individual. Although these claims are true, it implies that the care provider must only be responsive to the one cared for. However, one can be extremely responsive to the needs of an individual and still not provide high quality care. As Marian Barnes (2012) observes, "There is much that is called care that is not care" (p. 7). For example, if someone was hungry and I provided them with candy, there is certainly some level of care at work. The one receiving the care may be extremely pleased with receiving the candy. However, if I had provided a healthy nutritious meal to someone who is hungry, such an act would demonstrate a higher standard of care if generalized knowledge is taken into consideration. I would be bringing generalized knowledge of health and nutrition to the caring relationship. The significant point is that in every caring action, although the apparent phenomenon engages two people, there is usually an unspoken third party to the relationship: social and scientific evidence informing what constitutes good care. This describes the generalized knowledge of technical professionalism.

Like concrete knowledge, generalized knowledge can have propositional elements but it is also consists of "know-how." As previously described, propositional knowledge involves what are commonly referred to as facts justified by reliable evidence such as the consumption of high levels of cholesterol is associated with risk for heart disease or not smoking will prolong your life. Reliable evidence can be empirical in terms of repeated observation or the result of scientific investigation. In addition to propositional knowledge, generalized knowledge consists of "know-how" or the mental and physical skill to perform certain activities that take time and attention to learn. For example, the know-how can describe the skills necessary for flying an airplane, gourmet cooking, or teaching a college course in philosophy. Propositional knowledge and know-how exist in malleable categories and ranges of difficulty. Some skills take years to learn and others can be learned quickly. Some information is simple and easy to grasp and other information is complex and requires years of study.

Effective care requires the acquisition of generalized knowledge. This generalized knowledge is acquired not as a static bounded entity but as knowledge to be put to use with fine-tuned concrete knowledge. The psychologist learns about patterns of harmful human behavior not for the sake of learning a body of content knowledge but to put that understanding in interaction with concrete local knowledge in service of the patient. This is true of all care. The one caring brings to a relationship knowledge and experience that is not fixed but must come into engagement with the concrete knowledge of the one cared for. Thus generalized knowledge is crucial to caring activity.

Philosopher John Dewey (as cited in Boydston, 2008) offers a dynamic structure of inquiry that is particularly useful for considering the generalized knowledge necessary for care and its relationship to local knowledge. In particular his notions of habit, inquiry, and deliberation frame an epistemology that is nimble and open ended leaving room for interacting with what I have described as concrete knowledge. Dewey rejects passive spectator theories of knowledge in favor of an active theory of inquiry. In *The Quest for Certainty*, Dewey describes, "Our main attempt will be to show how the actual procedures of knowledge, interpreted after the pattern formed by experimental inquiry, cancel the isolation of knowledge from overt action" (Boydston, 1988b, p. 38). Dewey views inquiry as a human response that seeks resolution to dissonance: "Inquiry is the controlled or directed transformation of an indeterminate situation into one that is so determinate in its constituent distinctions and relations as to convert the elements of the original situation into a unified whole" (Boydston, 1991, p. 108). For Dewey, inquiry is animated by transactions individuals have with their environment. As Larry Hickman (1998) describes,

> Inquiry, and the theory of inquiry, were in Dewey's view among the most important tools at our disposal for learning to live together in ways that take into account the constraints of our environing conditions, as well as the full range of human needs and aspirations. (p. 186)

Knowledge production through inquiry is an acquired habit.

For Dewey, habits are acquired and open ended structures. As he describes, "The essence of habit is an acquired predisposition to *ways* or modes of response, not to particular acts except, as under special conditions, these express a way of behaving" (Boydston, 1988a, p. 32). Dewey (1966) describes inquiry as consisting of habits, or more accurately, chains or interconnections of habits (p. 390). The concept of habituation is dynamic for Dewey as every experience serves to modify the framework of the habit: "The basic characteristic of habit is that every experience enacted and undergone modifies the one who acts and undergoes, while this modification affects, whether we wish it or not, the quality of subsequent experiences" (Boydston, 2008, p. 18). Accordingly, knowledge is an indispensable outgrowth of every experience if we are open to the opportunity to learn. If not, our habits can become sedimented and lack growth potential. Tove Pettersen (2008) discusses something akin to a habit when she describes *care-cognition* as a learned ability of social responsiveness that mixes cognitive and emotional elements (p. 52).

For Dewey (Boydston, 2008), inquiry is a habit that all human beings should embrace as a response to solving life's challenges and conflicts. Generalized knowledge is acquired not to sit on a shelf but to be applied and adapted to given situations. However, the skills of adaptation should be considered and valued as important generalized knowledge as well. For example, listening skills qualify as generalized knowledge and they are habits of adaptation. Dewey's work suggests that the skilled professional is one who has the generalized knowledge of a given field as well as the skills of adaptation. The physician needs to know disease but also acquire the know-how to elicit information from the patient in order to understand the patient's context and condition. These are both forms of generalized knowledge.

Concrete and generalized knowledge are both needed for effective responsive care. Deweyan philosophy is also useful for the integration of concrete and generalized knowledge. Dewey defined moral deliberation as "a dramatic rehearsal (in imagination) of various competing lines of action" (Boydston, 1988a, p. 132). Such dramatic rehearsals are context-driven scenario explorations. In other words, Dewey's notion of deliberation can be understood as where concrete knowledge meets generalized knowledge in service of caring courses of action. Deliberation is also an appropriate term because although it can be undertaken by an individual, deliberation can connote a group effort including the one-cared for in the conversation.

To summarize, one must know how to care for someone as well as know a great deal about the one cared for in order to deliver rich and competent care. Taken together, the significance of concrete and generalized knowledge places a substantial demand on the caregiver to pursue knowledge. Fine tuning care for quality brings us to consider assessment. Furthermore, the negotiation between generalized and concrete care in a robust responsive care has implications beyond the actions of individuals directly involved in delivering care. Social and political institutions responsible for policies and practices regarding care have the same demands for a two-source approach to the knowledge necessary for competent care. Poverty, migration, and violent conflict require the theoretical and general knowledge gleaned from history and experience as well as the local knowledge that comes from the circumstances of individuals and communities to make effective caring decisions. For example, in "Global Care, Local Configurations—Challenges to Conceptualizations of Care," geography and migration scholar, Parvati Raghuram (2012) contends that contemporary migration literature tends to describe care in fairly homogenous terms. She claims that in reality, "The provision of care is differentially embedded in cultural, political and economic formations such as the family, the market, the state and the community sector in different countries" (p. 156). In very simple terms, aid and policies that may help one group of migrants may not be effective elsewhere. Raghuram is describing the negotiation between generalized and concrete care.

ASSESSING CARE

If caring is truly based on being responsive to the one cared-for then feedback is crucial to the one caring. The motivation to authentically care should include a desire to know if the care given is effective and how it can be made better. Assessment practices are an important mechanism for organized feedback. Based on the overlapping two-source model of caring knowledge offered above, assessment of care must include generalize and concrete elements. For example, one can offer a set of assessment questions for each. In service of concrete knowledge, an overarching question is whether the caregiver understood and responded to the needs and particular context of the one cared for. The one cared for is the primary arbiter of such concrete assessment. Other questions can also be directed at generalized knowledge, such as: "Did the caregiver know about all the options available?" and "Was the caregiver skilled at the care they delivered?"

By suggesting that education institutions should adopt care as a central value and focus, Noddings (2005) provides one context for assessing a two-source model of knowledge for care as described above. She is explicit in claiming that schools should be held accountable for what they educate (p. xiii), but believes that care should be at the heart of that accountability. Noddings (2005) introduces the value of choice in responsive caring. Depending on the context, if one is not given choices then it is difficult to view the one providing care as responsive rather than paternalistic. In terms of schools in the United States, Noddings (2005) claims,

> In keeping with the theme of responsiveness, teachers and students should stay together by mutual consent, and no student should be forced to stay with

> a teacher he or she hates or fears. I am arguing that it is important for families to have a choice between broadly different approaches to education, but if a child is miserable with a teacher whose approach seemed at first theoretically compatible, a change should be made. (p. xvii)

Choice of instructor and methodology according to Noddings (2005) can be a point of assessment when considering the effectiveness of caring in education. However, it is not the only criteria for assessment. Noddings (2005) further argues that individual "caring teachers listen and respond differentially to students" (p. 15). More specifically, "a faithful caring relation allows students to select and affirm their own interests after initial exposure" (p. 37). Noddings is suggesting that in a caring environment instructors are responsive to the content interests of the student. Setting aside the radical departure from established education structures that Noddings offers, one can see assessment criteria for educative care emerging from the idea of student autonomy and choice in the learning process. Questions regarding how instructors assist students pursue their intellectual curiosity can reveal one aspect of their effective care. The critical source for this assessment is the student, the one cared for.

One can readily see the pitfalls of bracketing responsive knowledge as the only criteria for care in the example above. Equally important to the responsive knowledge is the generalized knowledge derived from science and society. An effective teacher has generalized skills and knowledge that are significant to the learning experience such as communication skills, understanding developmentally appropriate pedagogical techniques as well as discipline specific content and methodologies. None of these are developed out of specific attention to the student but are adapted for the benefit of individual student learning. Noddings (2005), who spent many years as a math instructor, values the teaching of math and acknowledges the general need for quantitative literacy although she thinks it can be modified depending upon interest (p. 159). Because the history of education in the United States has been rigidly content-based, Noddings' critique focuses on responsiveness to concrete student circumstances. Nevertheless, the need for generalized knowledge in order to be effective is also present. The critical source for this generalized knowledge assessment is not the student but peers, independent observers, and evaluators who can measure whether the instructor has adequate content knowledge and teaching skill.

To omit assessing either the ability to engage concrete or generalized knowledge results in an incomplete picture of the professional teacher as such an omission misrepresents any professional. All work is marked by generalized skill and knowledge that has to be adapted to particular circumstances and individuals. Unfortunately, the notion of professional skill commonly relies on a few isolated variables of generalized knowledge. Medical professionals are valued for their diagnostic skill and biomedical knowledge. University professors are valued for their depth of discipline knowledge. Auto mechanics are valued for their ability to perform particular repairs. Lawyers are valued for their legal knowledge and analytical skills. Clearly, in each case the technical skills and knowledge are essential to the proficiency of these professionals. Furthermore, deeper technical specialization often receives additional social and economic valorization such as in the higher compensation and prestige of the surgeon, the managerial accountant, or the trial lawyer. However, what has been suggested here is that there is more to the story of professional competency than the generalized knowledge of technical specialization. Equally significant to technical skill for all professionals is their ability to effectively interact with others in a caring relationship. Interpersonal skills do not receive the same attention or explicit value as other skills. The amount of time spent on interpersonal proficiency in medical school, auto mechanics training, or law school is dwarfed by the quantity spend on technical training. However, social intelligence is not just a "social nicety" but contributes to what is understood as a proficient professional—a signifier element of general knowledge that should be assessed and maintained.

Health care provides a good example regarding the value of enlarged notions of professionalism because significant data on the experience of care has been collected. For example, in one large study, individuals who perceived empathy in their therapeutic interactions were correlated to shorter durations and less severity of common infectious diseases (Rakel et al., 2011). In another study, patient perception of physician empathy was a correlative determinant of overall evaluation of the medical experience even when treatment involved surgery, in which a high degree of technical skill is required (Steinhausen et al., 2014). Robust caring relationships can contribute to the range and depth of knowledge available to the medical professional (Hamington, 2012). The argument here is not that caring (based on concrete knowledge) supersedes technical skills (based on generalized knowledge) but that care cannot be disentangled from a complete understanding of professional competency. Any assessment of professional competency must include both.

Furthermore, an expansive definition of professional includes care, evaluation and feedback, which should be viewed as desirable if not mandatory. Professional competence is not static as in the achievement of a degree but dynamic and in constant need of fine tuning to maintain competency. The notion of ongoing professional education is well established in terms such as continuing professional education (CPE) or continuing professional development (CPD) such as understood among lawyers as continuing legal education (CLE). However, these terms refer to upkeep of generalized knowledge. Maintenance of concrete knowledge and the skills of acquiring it requires greater vigilance and ongoing effort in terms of seeking continuous feedback and responding to that feedback. If one cares about caring, then one should work to know if they are doing it well.

Barbara Brewer and Jean Watson (2015) describe the administration of the Watson Caritas Patient Score feedback instrument to over one thousand patients across a number of hospitals as a means to provide information regarding caring experiences. The instrument provides respondents with the opportunity to rate their care in five dimensions:

1. Deliver my care with loving-kindness.
2. Meet my basic human needs with dignity.
3. Have helping and trusting relationships with me.
4. Create a caring environment that helps me to heal.
5. Value my personal beliefs and faith, allowing for hope.

The instrument also offers an opportunity for an open-ended question regarding experiences that were caring or uncaring. Brewer and Watson (2015) find the data collected valid, reliable, and useful (p. 626). Although this is a positive step in valuing the concrete knowledge of those cared for in evaluative feedback, it also demonstrates some of the challenges and limitations of assessing responsive care. The data were generalized to hospitals and care units. Such analytical breakdown has utility, yet care is individually experienced and so the more challenging task of collecting and analyzing the caring practices of specific health care professionals is needed to improve professional behavior. In addition, the authors understandably referred to the data as "subjective experience" of the patient (Brewer & Watson, 2015, p. 626). For example, the authors describe, "To shift the focus from objective, problem-oriented criteria and measures that address the status quo, this study, grounded in caring science, represents an expanded framework for healthcare and subjective outcomes, guided by authentic human-to-human caring and assessing core variables of patient experiences of caring" (Brewer & Watson, 2015, p. 623). Granting that the experience was indeed subjective, if we consider care in terms of personal experience and perspective, the term implies a value judgment whereby so-called objective measures are somehow superior and more reliable. What I am suggesting is that we cannot understand what it is to be an effective professional without assessing responsiveness through the leveraging of both concrete and generalized knowledge.

SUMMARY SUGGESTION: A FRAMEWORK FOR EVALUATION OF PROFESSIONAL COMPETENCY

Given what has been argued for so far, I suggest a general structure for the evaluation of professional competency. Note that I am not specifying, "care" in the title because I am claiming that all professionals should have an element of care built into their work.

Broad Elements for Evaluation of Professional Competency

- Evaluation of Generalized Knowledge
  - Proficiency and knowledge in the field
  - Ability to adapt and communicate generalized knowledge
- Responsive skills (i.e., active listening, attentiveness)
- Evaluation of Concrete Knowledge
  - Understanding of individual cared for (i.e., patient, student, customer, etc.)
  - Understanding of context of the one cared for including, when appropriate, significant relationships affected

This is a very simple evaluation framework that reflects the two-source model of caring knowledge presented above.

CONCLUSION: THE NECESSITY OF RESPONSIVE EVALUATION

Although the above summary suggestion indicates the categories needed to assess caring professionalism, the method of gathering information for evaluation must be appropriate to capture the numerous relationships and tacit knowledge that constitutes concrete knowledge. The methods of *responsive evaluation*, an approach to evaluation developed by Robert Stake (Abma & Stake, 2001), appear particularly well suited to gather the kind of feedback needed to assess the utilization of concrete and generalized knowledge of the professional engaged in caregiving because of the extensive attention devoted to individuals and relationships. Responsive evaluation shares the valorization of two significant theoretical qualities with care ethics: particularism and relationality. Both of these qualities can be found in this concluding statement from an article on situational evaluation of educators by Stake and Cisneros-Cohernour (2000):

> We have discussed the evaluation of teaching with an emphasis on the context of work, the multidimensionality of competence, and the uniqueness of individual faculty members. These qualities, plus emphasis on personal intentionality and empathic understanding, have been common aspects of naturalistic, phenomenological, and ethnographic studies of teaching. Inquiry methods used in such studies have a potential for improving the quality of appraisal efforts. (p. 67)

In terms of particularism, both care ethics and responsive evaluation stress the significance of context. In this regard, both approaches challenged their fields in regard to objective positivism.

According to Stake (2014), "Responsive evaluation emphasizes a diversity of perspectives and an experiential portrayal of evaluand quality" (p. 448). Visse, Abma, and Widdershoven (2012) describe responsive evaluation as, "a dialogical process aimed at reaching mutual understanding between stakeholders on the object of evaluation. Consensus about the subject is not necessary, but mutual understanding is" (p. 98). Care ethics is founded on a relational ontology and epistemology that places the relationship as the central unit of meaning rather than abstract understanding of moral action. Accordingly, caring professionalism requires an assessment that valorizes relational experience. Abma (2005) characterizes responsive evaluation as grounded in social constructivist view of epistemology whereby humans are active agents in knowledge creation (p. 392). To conduct responsive evaluation effectively, evaluators actively embed themselves in the social dynamics of the evaluated community:

> In a responsive evaluation evaluator roles include those of interpretator, educator, facilitator and Socratic guide. As interpretator the evaluator has to endow meanings to issues. The role of educator refers to the creation of understanding by explicating various experiences to involved groups. Facilitator refers to the organization of the dialogue and the creation of required conditions. As Socratic guide the evaluator will probe into taken for granted ideas, final truths and certainties, and bring in new perspectives. (Abma, 2005, p. 392)

In particular, Visse, Abma, and Widdershoven (2015) have emphasized the democratic and participatory aspects of responsive evaluation that attends to the relative power and privilege dynamics within evaluated groups. Visse, Abma, and Widdershoven claim, "Responsive evaluators are not judges, but facilitate a deliberation process where authority is shared, where participants are supported in voicing their concerns and perspectives and are subsequently connected to political efforts" (p. 17). This is the kind of analysis that addresses the intricacies of complex human relationships. Responsive evaluations' relational approach can assess the ability of professionals to adapt generalized knowledge to particular individuals, as well as whether professionals are skilled at acquiring concrete knowledge. In other words, responsive evaluation is a form of caring inquiry. The evaluator immerses themselves in the relationships of care because that is the best way to truly understand what is going on between individuals. The delivery of quality care is dynamic in its ongoing adaptation to needs, as well as new generalized knowledge. Therefore robust feedback such as that found in responsive evaluation is essential.

Ultimately, caring and responsive evaluation are both forms of relational inquiry (Abma & Stake, 2001, p. 20) that do not shy away from empathy and understanding, and neither should professionals engaged in care labor.

KEY CONCEPTS

- care ethics
- competency
- concrete knowledge
- epistemology of care
- generalized knowledge
- habit
- inquiry
- presence
- professionalism
- responsive evaluation
- responsive care
- tacit knowledge
- two-source model for caring knowledge

DISCUSSION QUESTIONS

1. The chapter asserts that effective or competent care engages both generalized knowledge, including know-how and competency in a particular field of study, as well as concrete knowledge, the knowledge of the particular individual to be cared for. Under what conditions might generalized and concrete knowledge overlap?
2. The author suggests that care ethics and responsive evaluation share a number of theoretical underpinnings. What are some particular practices or methods of responsive evaluation that demonstrate care?
3. This chapter proposes that professionalism be redefined to include the epistemological practices of care. What are some of the challenges to widespread acceptance and implementation of an expansive definition of professionalism that includes care?

REFERENCES

Abma, T. A. (2005). Responsive evaluation in health promotion: Its value for ambiguous contexts. *Health Promotion International, 20*(4), 391–397.

Abma, T. A., & Stake, R. E. (2001). Stake's responsive evaluation: Core ideas and evolution. *New Directions for Evaluation, 92,* 7–21.

Baart, A. J. (2002). The presence approach, an introductory sketch of a practice. *Texts of the Presence Research,* Actioma: CTU Utrecht, Netherlands.

Baart, A. J., & Vosman, F. (2011). Relationship based care and recognition part one: Sketching good care from the theory of presence and five entries. In C. Gastmans, C. Leget, & M. Verkerk (Eds.), *Care, compassion and recognition: An ethical discussion* (pp. 183–200). Leuven, Belgium: Peeters.

Barad, K. (2007). *Meeting the universe halfway: Quantum physics and the entanglement of matter and meaning.* Durham, NC: Duke University Press.

Barnes, M. (2012). *Care in everyday life: An ethic of care in practice.* Bristol, England: Policy Press.

Benerìa, L. (2008). The crisis of care, international migration, and public policy. *Feminist Economics, 14*(3), 1–21.

Benhabib, S. (1987). The generalized and the concrete other: The Kohlberg-Gilligan controversy and moral theory. In E. Kittay & D. Meyers (Eds.), *Women and moral theory* (pp. 154–177). Lanham, MD: Rowman and Littlefield.

Benner, P., & Phillips, S. S. (1994). *The crisis of care: Affirming and restoring caring practices in the helping professions.* Washington, DC: Georgetown University Press.

Brewer, B. & Watson, J. (2015). Caring science research: Criteria, evidence, and measurement. *JONA 45*(12), 622–627.

Bunting, M. (2016, March 18). Crisis of care: The essay. [Radio Broadcast]. Retrieved from http://www.bbc.co.uk/programmes/b0741jl8/

Boydston, J. A. (Ed.). (1988a). *John Dewey: The middle works, 1899–1924: Human nature and conduct* (Vol. 14, 1922). Carbondale, IL: Southern Illinois University Press.

Boydston, J. A. (Ed.). (1988b). *John Dewey: The later works, 1925–1953: The quest for certainty* (Vol. 4, 1929). Carbondale, IL: Southern Illinois University Press.

Boydston, J. A. (Ed.). (1991). *John Dewey: The later works, 1925–1953* (12th ed.). Carbondale, IL: Southern Illinois University Press.

Boydston, J. A. (2008). *John Dewey: The later works, 1925–1953* (13th ed.). Carbondale, IL: Southern Illinois University Press.

Code, L. (2015). Care, concern, and advocacy: Is there a place for epistemic responsibility? *Feminist Philosophy Quarterly, 1*(1), 1–20.

Dalmiya, V. (2002). Why should a knower care? *Hypatia, 17*(1), 34–52. Retrieved from http://www.jstor.org/stable/3810580

Dewey, J. (1966). *Democracy and education.* New York, NY: Free Press.

Engster, D. (2007). *The heart of justice: Care ethics and political theory.* New York, NY: Oxford University Press.

Engster, D. (2015). *Justice, care, and the welfare state.* New York, NY: Oxford University Press.

Gilligan, C. (2011, June 21). *Carol Gilligan* [Interview]. Retrieved from http://ethicsofcare.org/carol-gilligan/

Hamington, M. (2004). *Embodied Care: Jane Addams, Maurice Merleau-Ponty and feminist ethics.* Urbana: University of Illinois Press.

Hamington, M. (2012). Care ethics and corporeal inquiry in patient relations. *International Journal of Feminist Approaches to Bioethics, 5*(1), 52–69.

Hamington, M. (2015). Politics is not a game: The radical potential of care. In D. Engster & M. Hamington (Eds.), *Care ethics and political theory* (pp. 272–292). New York, NY: Oxford University Press.

Hamington, M. (2016). Empathy and Care Ethics. In H. Maibom (Ed.), *Routledge handbook of philosophy of empathy* (pp. 264–272). New York, NY: Routledge, forthcoming.

Held, V. (2006). *The ethics of care: Personal, political, and global.* New York, NY: Oxford University Press.

Hickman, L. A. (1998). Dewey's theory of inquiry. In L. A. Hickman (Ed.), *Reading Dewey: Interpretations for a postmodern generation* (pp. 166–186). Bloomington, IN: Indiana University Press.

Kittay, E. F. (2015). A theory of justice as fair terms of social life given our inevitable dependency and our inextricable interdependency. In D. Engster & M. Hamington (Eds.), *Care ethics and political theory* (pp. 51–71). New York, NY: Oxford University Press.

Kittay, E. F., & Feder, E. K. (2003). *The subject of care: Feminist perspectives on dependency.* Totowa, NJ: Rowman and Littlefield.

Klaver, K., & Baart, A. (2011). Attentiveness in care: Towards a theoretical framework. *Nursing Ethics, 18*(5), 686–693.

Klaver, K., Elst, E., & Baart, A. (2015). Demarcation of the ethics of care as a discipline: Discussion article. *Nursing Ethics 21*(7), 755–765.

Noddings, N. (1984). *Caring: A feminine approach to ethics and moral education.* Berkeley, CA: University of California Press.

Noddings, N. (1988). Schools face 'crisis in caring. *Education Week, 8*(14), 32.

Noddings, N. (2002) *Starting at home: Caring and social policy.* Berkeley, CA: University of California Press.

Noddings, N. (2005). *The challenge to care in schools* (2nd ed.). New York, NY: Teachers College Press.

Noddings, N. (2010). *The maternal factor: Two paths to morality.* Berkeley, CA: University of California Press.

Pettersen, T. (2008). *Comprehending care: Problems and possibilities in the ethics of care.* Lanham, MD: Lexington Books.

Polanyi, M. (1966). *The tacit dimension.* Gloucester, MA: Peter Smith.

Puig de la Bellacasa, M. (2010). Ethical doings in naturecultures. *Ethics, Place and Environment, 13*(2), 151–169.

Puig de la Bellacasa, M. (2011). Matters of care in technoscience: Assembling neglected things. *Social Studies of Science, 41*, 85–106.

Puig de la Bellacasa, M. (2012). Nothing comes without its world: Thinking with care. *The Sociological Review, 60*(2), 197–216.

Pulcini, E. (2016). What emotions motivate care? *Emotion Review,* 1–8.

Raghuram, P. (2012), Global Care, Local Configurations—Challenges To Conceptualizations Of Care. *Global Networks, 12*(2), 155–174.

Rakel, D., Barrett, B., Zhang, Z., Hoeft, T., Chewning, B., Marchand, L., & Scheder, J. (2011). Perception of empathy in the therapeutic encounter: Effects on the common cold. *Patient Education and Counseling, 85*(3), 390–397.

Reinders, H. (2010). The importance of tacit knowledge in practices of care. *Journal of Intellectual Disability Research, 54*(Suppl. 1), 28–37.

Robinson, F. (1999). *Globalizing care: Ethics, feminist theory, and international relations.* Boulder, CO: Westview Press.

Robinson, F. (2011). *The ethics of care: A feminist approach to human security.* Philadelphia, PA: Temple University Press.

Sevenhuijsen, S. (1998). *Citizenship and the ethics of care: Feminist considerations on justice, morality and politics.* New York, NY: Routledge.

Slote, M. (2007). *The ethics of care and empathy.* New York, NY: Routledge.

Slote, M. (2010). *Moral sentimentalism.* New York, NY: Oxford University Press.

Stake, R. (2014). Information science and responsive evaluation. *E–Learning and Digital Media, 11*(5), 443–450.

Stake, R., & Cisneros-Cohernour, E. J. (2000). Situational evaluation of teaching on campus. *New Directions For Teaching And Learning, 83,* 51–72.

Steinhausen, S., Ommend, O., Thûmb, S., Lefering, R., Thorsten, K., Neugebauer, E., & Pfaff, H. (2014). Physician empathy and subjective evaluation of medical treatment outcome in trauma surgery patients. *Patient Education and Counseling, 95*(1), 53–60.

Tronto, J. C. (1993). *Moral boundaries: A political argument for an ethic of care.* New York, NY: Routledge.

Tronto, J. C. (2013). *Caring democracy: Markets, equality, and justice.* New York, NY: New York University Press.

Verducci, S. (2000). A moral method? Thoughts on cultivating empathy through method acting. *Journal of Moral Education, 29,* 87–99.

Visse, M., Abma, T. A., & Widdershoven, G. A. M. (2012). Relational responsibilities in responsive evaluation. *Evaluation and Program Planning, 35,* 97–104.

Visse, M., Abma, T. A., & Widdershoven, G. A. M (2015). Practising political care ethics: Can responsive evaluation foster democratic care? *Ethics and Social Welfare* [online publication].

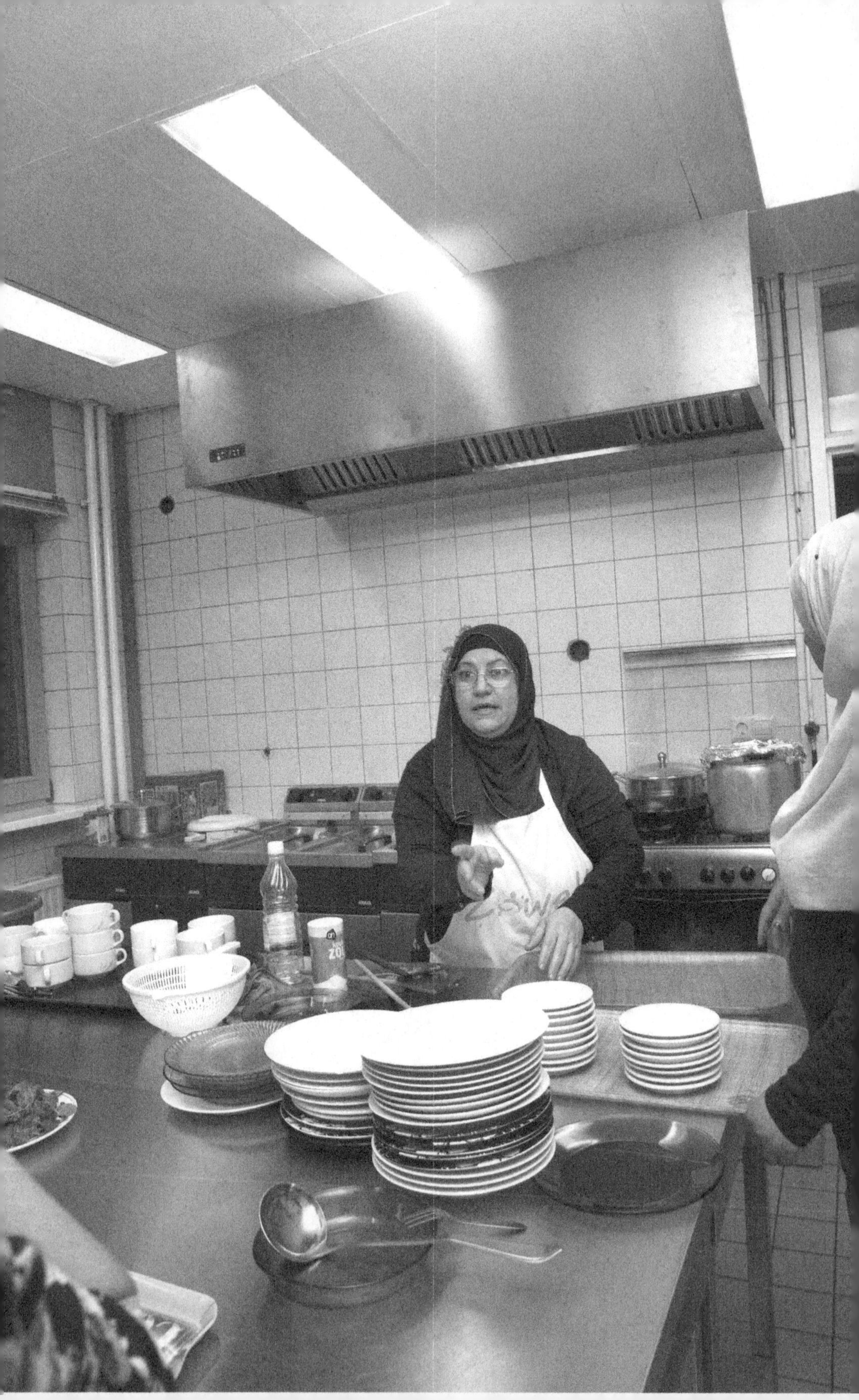

CHAPTER 2

THE ART OF UNDERSTANDING

Karin Dahlberg
Linnaeus University, Sweden

Science manipulates things and gives up living in them.
—Merleau-Ponty (1989b, p. 159)

The thesis of this chapter is that *understanding* is a key phenomenon in caring practice, as well as in all kinds of investigations of care. In caring science research, or projects evaluating caring practice, the goal is to better understand some aspects of health and caring; that is, we want to understand how the care works and if it improves health and life as it is supposed to. In order to reach this goal, we need to understand the persons for whom the care is intended. We need to understand if and how the care is embracing the care commitments, for example, if health care supports the patients' health processes, which includes the experience of well-being and the capacity of managing one's minor and life projects. Especially the latter is also valid for social care.

Understanding in this context is related to something different and more than what a person thinks or says about the care. It is about what and how the care meaningfully changes the person's life situation, with a focus upon health. Consequently it is both essential and a challenge to understand how the care is for the person who is a patient or client, that is, how the care is experienced and lived by them. Such interest also means to be

Evaluation for a Caring Society, pages 51–79

aware of how misunderstanding happens. It means recognizing when we do not reach another human and her/his experiential world, that is, the lifeworld, our common background for understanding our world and at all having a world.

Health care has had a tendency of caring paternalism, where the patient or client is a passive receiver of care. Nowadays it is more likely that it has turned over to the other side with the neo-liberal emphasis on patients or clients as customers, which has a too strong emphasis on human and economic rationality. As an alternative, lifeworld-led care and research balances the opposites and supports the rationale of existence. Such care is always on the patient's side, respecting both existential vulnerability and patient agency. Understanding a person in such a way has a profound ethical meaning. Consequently, all kinds of research and evaluation of care will benefit from a thorough consideration of what lifeworld-led approaches have to offer.

THE EVERYDAY ATTITUDE OF UNDERSTANDING

In many situations, in research as well as in caring practice, we often and easily say, "I understand." All daily living is built upon such for granted-taken assumption that we do understand each other. Most often we probably do. If I ask my friend if she wants to take a walk with me and she says that she would like to but that she has some student essays to go through first, I might feel a bit disappointed. But I understand what she means by what she says—that she will take a walk with me, but not right now.

Even in health or social care we assume that we do understand each other when we talk about everyday matters. We assume that professionals talk with, listen to, and understand the patients. We hear professionals who declare that they emphasize the importance of openly understanding their patients or clients and that the care is built upon this very important ambition of understanding the persons who are patients. However, we can easily find descriptions by persons who express how they were not listened to, that they instead were ignored and objectified by the professionals. Also in research or other investigations of care, openness to the patients or clients and their perspectives is described as an important feature, and the goal is often described as democratic. We easily find evaluation projects that seem to have high goals, expecting to reveal the effects of treatments for the persons in focus or to discover their experiences in one or another way, but which nevertheless only measure what is measurable and at the same time ignore such phenomena that are really important for the persons, their health, their lives and other existential aspects that are not measureable. An example of such a phenomenon may be the awkward feeling of *unhomelikeness* that can occur when one is ill (see below). Likewise we can find qualitative inquiry that has failed its purpose. Reading interview transcripts we find interviewers not listening at all to their respondents but following their own agenda, steering the interview in a direction far from the interviewees' experiences. Looking at these events we can conclude that neither caring professionals nor investigators have understood—even if they themselves think that they have. I do not think that investigators try to hide the truth or that care professionals in general are following a hidden agenda. Instead I believe that understanding is a much more complex and even somewhat enigmatic phenomenon. It is existentially basic and in that sense a very simple phenomenon, and at the same time it has these complicated and difficult meanings that make it hard to really grasp and describe comprehensively. Questions arise: "What is understanding?," "How do we know that we have understood?," "Is it really possible to fully understand the experiences of another?," "How is it to be understood?," and "How can understanding be improved in the health care context?"

AIM AND METHOD

In this paper, consisting of two sections, my aim is to explore the phenomenon of *understanding*, without trying to avoid the depth of it, in order to see its ethical role in health and social care. The first section is a phenomenological analysis of understanding. I want to show how phenomenology outlines a philosophy of science that can challenge contemporary comprehension of existential conditions that are blurred by dualism and other reductionistic controversies. In this section the aim is to explore the phenomenon of understanding as openness to the lifeworld and how it is at all possible to understand a fellow human being. I address phenomenology (and hermeneutics) as a philosophy of in-between and how such an approach can illuminate the phenomenon of understanding (Dahlberg, Dahlberg, & Nyström 2008).

In the second section the intention is to use the outcome of the philosophical analysis to show how a thoughtful reflection of understanding has implications for both health and social care practice and investigations in these areas. I give examples of how understanding benefits from an open attitude to the lifeworld, with which professionals can better understand how existential dimensions are involved even in simple situations. I also present ideas of how investigations can be far more effective and show better evidence with lifeworld-led and verbal (and nonverbal) explorations instead of just diving deeper into the world of numbers.

Basically my own experience is health care practice and research. Therefore my illustrations come from that area. However, I am seriously interested in covering also social care, which is an area that I have explored theoretically as well as in health care research.

As a supporting strategy for the reader to see from where I understand the issue of understanding I will first, briefly, clarify my standpoints in relation to health and care as well as in phenomenology. At the same time this confession serves as an ontological and epistemological background for the analysis of understanding.

CARING FOR EXISTENTIAL VULNERABILITY

As existential philosophers have explored and debated, the only thing we know for sure is that our life will end. We do not know when or how, only that it will end. Everything else is uncertain. The existential uncertainty is hard to deal with and many may try to ignore it. Within our modern society we have built numerous strategies to forget about the finitude, and illness is sometimes that which reminds us of our existential conditions. Illness has the power of breaking down one's world, redefining it from being an experience of at-homeness and security to an experience of unhomelikeness and uncertainty, where one's life becomes strange and out of control (Svenaeus, 2001; Jingrot & Rosberg, 2008; van Wijngaarden, Leget, & Goossensen, 2015). Illness displays the vulnerability that lies in the tension between humans as, on the one hand, biologically and sociologically determined and *only being*, and, on the other hand, non-determined, free, and *becoming*. Caring science, my research context, is placed in-between these positions, recognizing both the determination and the freedom.

Vulnerability is often seen as human weakness and thus something negative, but it is important to include even the positive side of this existential condition. Heidegger, Merleau-Ponty, Ricoeur, and Sartre are philosophers who, among many others within continental philosophy, have analysed human existence. They have elegantly revealed how we all are limited by some aspects that we were born into, and which we can never completely free us from, but how we at the same time always have possibilities to overcome some definiteness and, in an existential way, also define ourselves and others, how we shape our own and others' lives, as well as how we are defined and shaped by others. Not least in caring science research we can see various descriptions of how illness turns out to be a wake-up call for a more existentially authentic living. We have found examples of how health can be experienced stronger, more present, even in states that are characterized by severe illness (Dahlberg & Segesten, 2010).

It is the responsibility of health (and social) care professionals to appreciate and respond to the existential vulnerability and how it presents itself in the individual person. Care professionals have to act in response to every patient or client as an existential being that is both being and becoming. With a lifeworld approach all care is established on an understanding of health, in addition to something biological, as it is experienced in the context of everyday life. In such an approach, health means a sense of well-being as well as a capacity to *realize one's minor and major life projects.* In health care, all caring efforts should support patients' health processes so that even if illness is a fact, one can be well, feel good, and can do that which is important to do, on an everyday basis or in the longer run. Even in social care the focus must be on well-being as well as a capacity to run one's life in a positive, creative and constructive way. Supporting a person's health (and social) processes thus has a goal of *existential vitality,* which also includes a sense of *life-meaning* and *life-rhythm,* as well as of social relationships and the experience of *belongingness.* However, it is important to say that this theory is descriptive, not normative. It does not demand from anyone to find meaning every time or everywhere, but it demands from professionals to be openly understanding how these existential aspects, such as vitality, meaning and rhythm, present themselves in the patients or clients.

Consequently, the focus upon health and well-being is superior to the focus upon disease, illness or other forms of dysfunction. That is, all care (even social care) should be directed towards health as well-being and the capacity of running one's life projects. Even in situations when people live with severe and maybe life-threatening illness, the emphasis on lived health has a profound meaning, as it supports the vital forces in the person in care. Even in palliative situations and situations when professionals must relate to people with death wishes, a lifeworld approach to health with this described meaning is crucial (van Wijngaarden, Leget, & Goossensen, 2016). Such an approach unites the natural and human science perspectives on health and caring, since biological health is included in this approach, together with the notion of existential vitality, life-meaning and life-rhythm. It is such care that can connect with both definiteness and indefiniteness, and work in and with the tension between existential determination and freedom (Dahlberg, Todres, & Galvin, 2009; Dahlberg & Segesten, 2010; Ranheim, Kärner, & Berterö, 2012).

Lifeworld-led care has an existential power that can promote professionals who aim at strengthening patients' or clients' health processes and thereby balancing their efforts in relation to the human vulnerability. It is by lifeworld-led care that professionals can support persons who suffer from an overwhelming experience of not being able to live further in a decent way, as well as those who experience that their suffering means something good, something that helps them to better realize their life projects.

The focus upon existential vulnerability is valid also for the professionals themselves. If they are able to recognize their own vulnerability and respond to it in a professional and creative way, there is a strength with which they can apprehend others' suffering as well as their opportunities for a good life. Also, ethical stress in professionals is less likely to appear if care organisations adapt to lifeworld-led care and evaluation. And, it is within such an approach to care that I want to explore the art of understanding.

THE PHENOMENOLOGICAL APPROACH

As indicated above and for the purpose of this chapter, I do not separate between phenomenology and hermeneutics. My approach to understanding as a phenomenon is based within the so called continental school of philosophy where the characteristics of human existence form an ontology that is the origin for epistemology as well as methodology. Phenomenology is an approach that began with Husserl and was further developed by Merleau-Ponty, but which also includes thought patterns from other philosophers after Husserl, such as Heidegger, Gadamer, and Ricoeur whose work also is called hermeneutics.

It is not an easy task to work with Husserl's philosophy. As Merleau-Ponty (2002) also argues, Husserl never came to a once and for all clearly outlined conclusion and he is often depicted as the eternal beginner or the philosopher of infinite tasks (c.f. Natanson, 1973). Husserl's phenomenology is first and foremost a big gift to European philosophy. It consists of many large texts, of which some were posthumously published. The texts are impressively rich and with many extensions, but from the beginning to the end he wanted to describe the relationship between humans and that which we call our world. In order to address this huge problem he saw it necessary to encounter it from several different perspectives.1

In an analysis of phenomenology grounded in Husserl, another challenge is to involve ideas by Merleau-Ponty and not least by Heidegger and Gadamer. Without neglecting the huge discussion of the relationships between these philosophers' philosophy, I emphasize the ideas that unite them. Even if they have paved their own philosophical ways, to a great extent they follow some main patterns in Husserl. I maintain that they all relate to a profound understanding of humanity and existence as lifeworld, even when they do not use the concept. Gadamer (cf. 1976, 1995) does use this concept and he also clearly explores the idea in his thorough analyses of health (Gadamer, 1996). Heidegger (1998) describes being and how being is always related to time, in a way that unmistakably places him within lifeworld phenomenology, even if he is as unmistakably clear about a strong critique of Husserl, whom he thought was not paying enough attention to ontology. Merleau-Ponty, is the one who follows Husserl most closely and here I rely on his own statements (cf. 2002) as well as on the work by H. Dahlberg (2013) and her research of Merleau-Ponty's (2013) idea *flesh*.

As a conclusion, it is phenomenology as a broad, deep, and thorough philosophy of existence and knowledge development that I benefit from when I try to say something new and important about understanding and how this phenomenon is essential in care practise and in all kinds of investigations of care. In particular, as I see it, it is phenomenology as the *philosophy of in-between* that can unite care ethics with *the how* of evaluations of care.

SECTION 1: UNDERSTANDING IN THE PHILOSOPHY OF IN-BETWEEN

If there is one thing that must be said about phenomenology that connects all the main ideas and distinguishes this philosophy from all other modern ones, it is its fundamental focus upon *in-between*. When the rest of European philosophy makes up for a dispute on the question if existence is best explained through materialism or idealism, psychologism or empiricism, phenomenology offers a radical solution: It is neither the one side nor the other, the answer is in-between. When modern medicine and psychology describe humans as parts, consisting of body and psyche/soul, and when modern sociology prefers the societal perspective before the individual, phenomenology says that it is both. Phenomenology is clear: Existence is to be found in-between and it always moves between the different positions.

All through his writing, Husserl maintains that we can never understand existence or an aspect of it if we keep on working within dualism or other forms of strong dichotomies. The world of existence is not this simple, solid and never-changing reality that we take for granted in our natural attitude. Existence must be understood as co-constituted, Husserl emphasizes, it is always to be found within the relationship between ourselves and others, between ourselves and that which we call our world (c.f. 1970a, 1970b, 1973, 1977, 1998, 2000).[2]

In an early work, Merleau-Ponty (1995) discusses psychologism and empiricism. He concludes that even though they seem to be antithetical, both perspectives were born from the very same standpoint, namely dualism, and therefore they misunderstand our reality. Merleau-Ponty (1968) further progresses this central idea when he develops the ontology of flesh. He shows how it is not only the human body that can be understood as flesh, but being itself. In such understanding being cannot be approached at distance, as a scientist looks at an object of science through a microscope. Researchers questioning the world are themselves part of being, a being that consists of several layers or sides, a being that is never complete but always open, always changing, and it remains exposed to relationships that define and change it (Dahlberg, 2013).

THE WORLD OF PERCEPTION

Human existence is a world of perception. In our everyday life, most of the time we are actively engaged in the world by seeing, hearing, and touching. We are, in fact, engaged in the world already before we come aware of it. When I notice that I see a house, I have already seen a house, even if I only see the front of it. If I am waiting in a hospital for examination of my broken arm and a person in a white coat enters the room, I do not see "a person" in a "white coat," I see a physician. We are constantly moving towards an understanding of the world, and in this way we are constantly ahead of ourselves. This is what the phenomenological theory of intentionality is about.

As Husserl (e.g., 1973, 1998) states, intentionality can explain our relationships with others, the world, and the things that we use and that we see around us as the things, activity, and places that belong to and signify our world. In our daily living we are most often directed out from ourselves and to the world that we live and interact with. Intentionality is an endlessly ongoing bodily, sensing, perceptual, and understanding activity that structures that which we call lifeworld. Merleau-Ponty (1995), who took on the theory of intentional structures, cited Husserl by stating that "consciousness is consciousness of something" (p. 137) and by explaining how all experience is of the world. This means that perception has its "perceived," the wish its "wished for," the thought its "idea," anticipation has its "anticipated," and so on. Also Gadamer (1995) expresses how every existing "thing" has validity for us in its "givenness" (p. 244). Intentionality has to do with how things are given to us in experience, how we experience the things and how these things present themselves to us, how they are always meaningful for us and present themselves *as* something or other. We cannot even escape meaning; "Because we are in the world, we are *condemned to meaning*," as Merleau-Ponty (1995, p. xix, emphasis in original) puts it. And the process when meaning comes to be cannot be reduced to any -ism, for example to any side in a dualism, it happens in the in-between, which is in focus in a lifeworld approach.

Explicitly or implicitly, we understand the meaning of human action and the things that we use and see or in other ways experience around us as the things and places that belong to and signify our world. The reason that the experience is always a full one, that we see a house even if we only see the front side of it, is that it involves intentional horizons. And it is the same intentional event when we perceive other humans. It is the same givenness and the same intentional horizons that are in play. We see people around us without reflecting upon it. When I leave the airplane in Tokyo, not for a moment do I hesitate that what I see around me are other humans, even if this is my first time in Japan or Asia. In a hospital I immediately see professionals and patients. Husserl (cf. 1970b 1973, 1977, 1998) explains that every perception has a horizon belonging to it, a horizon that emerges with the act of perceiving. He calls these horizons *apperceptions* or *appresentations.* In every particular experience there is such an appresentation, which transcends the immediate given, and makes an existence in space and time possible, which our senses give to us as a whole. This is how understanding comes to be, and it is here we can find the explanations to why understanding happens or does not happen.

BODILY INTENTIONALITY

One main contribution to the theory of intentionality is when Merleau-Ponty (1989a, 1989b, 1995), based in Husserl's philosophy (2000; cf. Hamauzu, 2017), demonstrates how intentionality is embodied. It is not so much about "I think" but "I can." I am able to, when for example facing a house, move around it and see the other sides of it, and this ability affects my perception of the house. This has bearing on the understanding of others. If I walk on the street in my hometown and see a person coming against me, I immediately perceive my friend, Anna. And I also perceive her mood, that she is happy to see me. How do I know it is Anna and that she is happy? In fact, I see only some aspects of a full person and for example I definitely do not see her inside, her feelings or thoughts. My perception of Anna's happiness is not a rational conclusion. It is not that I think, "Aha, I see her particular form of the mouth and hand waves, I conclude that she is happy." It is a more immediate perception. Because I am and have a body, and because of my lived experience, I have access to my senses that contribute to the whole picture when I sense the other person and her mood.

Being bodily, we are already in a situation in the world before we come to reflect upon it, and it is this bodily being that is the existential humus from which understanding others can grow. The body is, as Merleau-Ponty chooses to phrase it, like the darkness in a theatre salon, needed for the spectacle on the stage to be seen. The body's role in our being and perception is seldom reflected upon, and there is a bodily engagement in the world that has already happened. It is afterwards that we can reflect upon this engagement, for example through the help of others (Merleau-Ponty, 1995, 1968; Dahlberg, 2013).

Let us stay some more with the question of how we perceive other persons and their emotions without having no direct access to their intentionality, and look at an approach that is often referred to as a way to understand others, namely empathy, which Husserl (cf. 1977, 2000) has analyzed. He describes how we, in empathy (*Einfülung*), form a *sphere of ownness* from which we understand *an-other,* as another self, an alter ego. Before Merleau-Ponty, Husserl (1977, 2000) denied that we exist just as physical bodies (*Körper*) and affirms that we also exist as animate organisms (*Leib*). The sphere of ownness serves as the bodily framework from which we understand another person. Just as our past experience with houses is the basis for anticipating a house when we see only the front of it, so do our own past experiences of ourselves (and others) provide an analogue for understanding others and their experiences. Interpreting Husserl's philosophy, Elliston (1977) explains that "the other is not given to me in exactly the same way I appear to myself... the similarity is mediated by a kind of *indirect* and counterfactual 'comparison': The other looks not the way I in fact look here but the way I would look if I were there" (p. 223, emphasis in original). Through experience and imagination and by comparing others' behavior, expressions, gestures, etc. with how one would think, feel, or be in the other person's place, one can come to understand something of them.

Merleau-Ponty (1991a) uses Husserl's term *Paarung* to explain how we encounter another, but emphasizes the bodily aspect of this meeting:

> It must be like a pairing (*Paarung*): A body encountering its counterpart in another body which itself realizes its own intentions and suggests new intentions to the self [*moi*]. The perception of others is the assumption of one organism by another.... The behavior of others conforms to my own intentions to such an extent, and designates a behavior which has so much meaning for me, that it is as though I assume it. (p. 43)

When we meet with others we see their behavior and recognize it as something that we also do or can do. When we recognize that the intentions lying behind others' behavior could be ours as well, we assume that emotions or intentions similar to ours underlie the behavior of others, even if it is about an experience that we do not have. Merleau-Ponty (1991a) gives us a compelling example:

> [I]n a fire, only the subject who is burned can feel the sensible sharpness of pain. But everything that the burn represents: the menace of fire, the danger for the well-being of the body, the significance of the pain, can be communicated to other people and felt by other people.... the intuition of the feeling (that which constitutes its essentials) is the same for the two consciousnesses. (p. 47)

A professional in health care may not have experienced particular illnesses but can still understand patients' suffering from not being well, for example not being able to move, work, or sleep without intense difficulty and great suffering.

It is against this background that we can understand Merleau-Ponty (1991b) when he says that "the other... is a generalized I," and that "my relation to myself is already generality" (p. 138). My understanding of the other is grounded in my understanding of myself, and vice versa. He furthermore states that: "There would be no others or other minds for me, if I did not have a body and if they had no body through which they slip into my field, multiplying it from within, and seeming to me prey to the same world, oriented to the same world as I" (1991b, p. 138). The reciprocity of intercorporeal communication, or "carnal intersubjectivity," as Merleau-Ponty (1987) also calls it, is not

> ... by a mind to a mind, but by a being who has body and language to a being who has body and language, each drawing the other by invisible threads like those who hold the marionettes—making the other speak, think, and become what he is but never would have been by himself. (p. 19)

In the quote, Merleau-Ponty (1987) displays how the existential co-constitution is embodied, how it belongs to the flesh of existence.

One of our prime ways of understanding the other in both research and caring practice is through language:

> There is one particular cultural object which is destined to play a crucial role in the perception of other people: language. In the experience of dialogue, there is constituted between the other person and myself a common ground: [M]y thought and his are interwoven into a single fabric. (Merleau-Ponty, 1995, p. 354)

We do not only belong to the same world, together we constitute the meaning of this world, of ourselves, and there is always more to a good meeting with another person than just two people exchanging information. Understanding grows both in the open conversation and in *the more* of it.

The intersubjective meeting gives rise to a situation where two body-subjects are being led by the meaning within and of the situation and conversation. Such a dialogue gives birth to memories and experiences that could have been forgotten a long time ago. Merleau-Ponty (1968) further describes this aspect of co-constitution by saying that:

> A genuine conversation gives me access to thought that I did not know myself capable of, that I was not capable of, and sometimes I feel myself followed in a route unknown to myself which my words, cast back by the other, are in the process of tracing out for me. (p. 13)

Such dialogue, which moves experiential borders, temporal as well as spatial, supports understanding.

THE NEED FOR BRIDLING

Together with others we form an existential corporeal field, which at the same time is a phenomenal field, that is, a field of meaning that asserts community (in the belongingness to the same world) and difference (in the uniqueness of every person). At the same time as everyone belongs to the same world, it is not the same for everyone. Even if we have much in common there is always something more, there is an element of uncertainty which we must attend to and approach other human beings with a careful curiosity, expecting to be surprised and see something unexpected and new. Because it is in this realm of uncertainty and otherness that misunderstanding grows.

The phenomenological analysis above gives a clear theoretical account of how understanding comes to be through our (bodily) intentionality. However, at the same time as understanding can be explained and mapped out for us as an ordinary event, we can also imagine how complicated every act of understanding can be and how many pitfalls there may be. All the time, misunderstanding, so to speak, lies in wait.

Understanding in general and our understanding of others in particular can never be guaranteed. Both Husserl (cf. 1970a, 1970b, 1973, 1977) and Merleau-Ponty (cf. 1968, 1989a, 1989b, 1995) granted this point by recognizing that the experiential horizons are open, that meaning is infinite, the future is never exhausted, and the process of understanding is never complete. Existence is marked by its in-betweenness. At the same time as we belong together, sharing the same world, the in-between can be seen as an open gap, a rift between ourselves and others. In order to realize all the opportunities of understanding others, which come with our being in a shared world, our ability of *pairing* and our way of being intentionally directed to our world through our bodies, we need to learn how to manage the gap between our own and others' experiential worlds, that is, we need to bridle the activity of understanding.

Originally, *bridling* was described in the context of research to replace the misunderstood concept of *bracketing* (Dahlberg, Dahlberg, & Nyström, 2008). Researchers should practise a disciplined interaction and communication with their phenomena and research participants, and bridle the event of understanding so that they do not take for granted that they understand even when they don't. Bridling prevents researchers from being carelessly or slovenly understanding, or in other words, that they quickly make definite what is indefinite (Dahlberg & Dahlberg, 2003). As such, bridling means an open and alert attitude of actively waiting for the phenomenon to show up and display itself and its meanings within the relationship with the researcher, which is a kind of "dwelling" with the phenomenon. The aim is to slow down the evolving understanding in order to see the phenomenon, the actual presentations as well as the ap-presentations, and all the different meanings that characterize something that is in focus. Instead of following the sometimes strong inputs from one's own pre-understanding and thus look backwards, one must re-direct one's perception forwards and onto the phenomenon. Instead of a quick decision of what something is or what seems to be discovered, the researcher must systematically, slowly, and carefully scrutinize the road to understanding.

Such an open attitude towards the event of understanding can also be applied in caring and social practise. The ambition to understand another person is sometimes explained as an ambition to put oneself in the other's shoes. This is not possible, as Husserl (1973), Merleau-Ponty (1995), and Gadamer (1995) argue. We can never free ourselves from our lifeworld, we always have our own experiential horizons from which we see and understand. The lifeworld that contributes with an opportunity of understanding others is also what sometimes hinders us from actually seeing others. The idea of bridling allows for our full experience to evolve and for a better understanding of the other.

Gadamer (1995) encourages us by emphasizing how all that is asked is "that we remain open to the meaning of the other." We must see "what is there" and not what we assume is there, we must separate our pre-understanding from the things themselves (p. 268–269). We must learn how not to follow the pre-understanding in a blind or deaf way, that we dwell with the meanings instead of quickly making decisions of what we see or hear in the other person. We have to be open for the otherness of existence to show itself, and we maybe have to actively look for "the alterity" as Gadamer (1995) puts it.

In a recent article (Todres, Galvin, & Dahlberg, 2014) we draw on the ethics by Levinas (1969) who unfolds what he refers to as *the infinity of otherness*. This can be further understood by Merleau-Ponty's (1968) analysis of the encounter with the other, which he says is characterized by "a partial coincidence," that is the other not just visible but also invisible; "... it is in making the other not only inaccessible but invisible for me that I guarantee his alterity" (p. 79). There is a gap in the understanding of the other, which means that the other is never fully understood but keeps her/his "otherness." If we want to understand what the other's smile means, not only to us but also for her/him, an understanding of the other's otherness is necessary, and the road there is bridling the on-going understanding.

In all understanding we have to be careful, and reflect not only on the meanings that we immediately see in the other person or the situation that we experience. We have to be open for the unexpected to come through, or in other words, to expect the unexpected, and to ask questions even when we think we already have the answers.

UNDERSTANDING ONESELF

Sometimes we think that understanding another is very different from understanding oneself, that while others are foreign subjects at least we know ourselves. This is a delusion.

We may be convinced that we know ourselves well; we know what we like or dislike, or what we want in our lives. However, a good talk with a friend or some meditative self-reflection might show something else and maybe change one's self-view. Psychotherapy builds on the idea that we do not know ourselves in that clear (self-evident) way we want to believe. A client in therapy is encouraged to stop for a while and, with support of the therapist, take a better look on oneself, for example from new perspectives, in order to understand oneself better. In a similar way a crisis, such as attracting some illness, losing a bodily function, or losing a job, make us existentially aware in a new way.

To understand another person and to understand oneself is essentially the same event, and involves the same mechanisms. In both instances understanding is based in the natural attitude, the stance when one takes for granted that what one sees is there. A word or even a glance from another person may change one's self-image. When one's self-image is even a little shaken, well, then one's view of the other also changes, and so on. Understanding is always in movement (Dahlberg, 2014; Dahlberg & Dahlberg, 2015).

CONCLUDING SECTION 1

It has been revealed how understanding operates in the in-between, how it is always moving between oneself and the world, between oneself and other persons. Understanding is always *on go*, ready to travel in one or other direction and hence there is also always the possibility for misunderstanding. As a starting point for the next section we can conclude that phenomenology provides us with essential knowledge of how understanding works. If we do not want to remain in the unreflective and taken for granted position of the so called natural attitude, we must cultivate the capacity of bridling the ongoing understanding in favor of a reflective and open attitude, to oneself, to others and to the world that we share. For all professionals in health and social care, practitioners as well as researchers and evaluators, it is of significant value to be aware of how the lived existential world works, how we all live in and through a world of intentional perception, where meanings come to be. Just to be open to the possibility of others' experiential worlds being surprisingly similar but also quite different from one's own, has a profound ethical meaning. The challenge is to empower understanding in such a way that the manifold of nuances of the lifeworld are displayed and come to play.

SECTION 2: LIFEWORLD-LED CARING PRACTICE AND EVALUATION

The doubleness of existence involves how we on the one hand share a common world and a common humanity and that on the other hand never can fully grasp all the meanings of the common world or humanity. If we want to realize the role of understanding in (social) caring practice we must admit both the generality and the particularity of this phenomenon, and let understanding move between the poles. We should not allow for polarisation of that which only seems to be opposite. Instead we must embrace the complexity of understanding, which in fact is founded in the complexity of existence, the intricate web of life, where understanding others is of vital significance. As if that is not enough difficult in general, understanding others who are patients or clients adds to the complexity. Understanding these others, whose main interest is to experience well-being and to go on with one's life, sometimes with severe illness or some dysfunction as a demanding companion, forms a particular field of meaning that requires of professionals to know how to carefully choose their way of acting.

To move comfortably in the unpaved field of in-between in health and social care and evaluation we can begin listening to Gadamer's (1995) advice, to first of all understand that we do not understand. Professionals have expert knowledge and sometimes long and substantial experience. We know a lot. But we do not know what this specific person here and now want to reveal to us. We do not know how s/he responds to illness or dysfunction, or what health, well-being and care mean to her/him. In order to encompass even such knowledge we must listen carefully to that person and see her/him in her/his context—even if what we see or hear is similar to or different from us, even if we expect a particular answer and receive a completely different one. Instead of resting safely and comfortably in our taken-for-granted understanding we must try hard to see even that which may seem unlikely, that which makes us surprised and sometimes puts us off. Listening and seeing in such a way, beginning in the awareness of not knowing, is a cornerstone of all kinds of care and evaluation, whether it is about finding the right care for the individual person or if it is about understanding the outcomes of given treatment or other steps taken.

It may seem to be an easy task. And it is. When someone cries out her/his anxiety over being diagnosed by an incurable disease, it is easy to say that we understand her/his feelings at that moment, being ready to support and comfort the person. And at the same time it is a difficult task, because we really do not know the meaning of this cry of anxiety. The patient or client may for example be an adult man coming from a culture where it is a male duty to support one's family, economically as well as socially. Being knocked down by severe illness might alter this person's whole life. The illness has already broken his body but will soon also break his whole existence. A professional who gets ready to comfort him at that moment will probably add to his burden, telling him that he now has become a poor man, a no-man.

To openly listen to the voice of the lifeworld is of immense significance. To begin with, such openness is about professionals' attitude and stance towards a patient, client or a participant in an evaluation. There must be a kind of unassuming, unpretentious and respectful position from which the professional can begin to probe the others and the lifeworld, to listen in different ways and ask questions that reveal more of the unknown. In such stance the doubleness and in-between perspective of understanding is obvious. We must always be aware that at the same time as we do understand, we do not understand. Such attitude is well described as the position of *here and now.* We always understand others, and we can very well understand differently, precisely *because* we are here and now. Presence here and now is thick of co-constituted meaning. It is in the moment of attention here and now that we can become intensely aware and see something new and unexpected. Cavalcante Schuback (2006) explains such open attitude as being a tourist in one's own hometown, where one sees the well-known in a different and new way, as if it is the first time one visits this town. It is an ethical demand to openly, attentively, and interestedly respond to patients, clients, or participants as persons, aiming at understanding them existentially, with their living contexts.

As professionals, we consequently try to find a good perspective, from which we can understand every patient or client, in care as well as in an investigation. We may benefit from an attitude when we unlearn taken-for-granted habits and instead adopt an attitude of not-knowing and alertness. The urge to choose such good a position, being close enough or distant enough, does not mean, as it may sound, to stand still. On the contrary it means to keep on moving, sensitively following the person that we want to understand, all the time being ready to ask new questions, or to offer some room for silence, for dwelling. It is about being actively alert, here and now.

Professionals who listen openly to the lifeworld, showing that they are trying to understand a patient, client, or a participant in an investigation, signal recognition, that s/he is worth listening to. In such an approach to the person, the existential vulnerability is also recognized and its full spectrum can be utilized. This is an instance which shows how understanding in all kinds of caring practice as well as in research, per definition, is about ethics.

HOW TO EMPOWER UNDERSTANDING—SOME EXEMPLARS

Professionals are humans and humans seek security. In general, we do not want to throw ourselves into the unknown. As Gadamer (1995) says, the event of openly understanding and entering the unknown means to risk or even lose oneself. It is an adventure to leave the comfortable zone where everything is familiar and well known and enter a journey which we do not know where it ends. However, this is what we must do if we want to sincerely understand a fellow human. This is what we must do if we want to encounter a person as a Thou and not as a foreign and distant object (Gadamer, 1995), or as simply another myself.

How then can professionals improve their ability of insiderness, an open and sensitive insight into a person's experiential domain, the lifeworld? How can they put themselves in play without feeling this as threatening? How can professionals develop their own humanity, a sensing, emotional and cognitive competence with which they can better understand others?

Ranheim (2011, Ranheim, Kärner, & Berterö, 2012) advocates that care professionals develop what she calls an *expanded awareness*, which is about cultivating and widening one's experiential horizons. Todres et al. (2014) are on the same line arguing that an ability of insiderness can only occur by the use of oneself rather than the application of already made knowledge in using a method (cf. Gadamer, 1995, 1996). One way of expanding one's awareness and enable understanding is to meet with other professionals in dialogue groups. To tell others of one's experiences and listening to others is inspiring and enriching, and may deepen one's way of understanding oneself or others. Sometimes just listening to oneself saying something loud can illuminate one's own feelings and reactions, and others' feelings, thoughts and reactions listening to it may also bring some new light on to a difficult situation.

In several clinical projects, Ekebergh (2007, 2009, 2011) and coworkers have developed a model for clinical reflection in nursing education. In groups of students, a university teacher and a nurse, the aim has been to enhance a deeper lifeworld-led understanding of caring with the patient and the lifeworld in focus. The students bring clinical narratives that are discussed and reflected upon with a foundation of caring science theory. The reflection takes place in dialogues, but also in nonverbal communication such as educational drama. Ekebergh (2007, 2009, 2011) maintains that lifeworld-led reflection, with the aim of developing caring knowledge, can never be simplified or discerned as an isolated method or technique, if the aim is to support an individual's growth of knowledge and to understand the otherness of others. That is why she prefers an open lifeworld approach. She also emphasizes the importance of keeping the groups small. Every student must have the experience of being recognized, which gives room for a parallel process, according to Ekebergh, who holds that the learning relationship and the caring relationship display similar features. According to Ekebergh (2007, 2009, 2011) and Berglund (2014), care is understood as a dialogical learning process. Similar ideas have been put forward by Halling (2006; Halling & Leifer, 1991,) in what he calls *dialogal research*, which may interest evaluators even more than the outcomes of care practice.

Patients can also be engaged in meetings focused upon care. Lindberg, Hörberg, Persson, & Edebergh, 2013a, 2013b, 2015) have reported a project where older patients were invited to team meetings, which substituted traditional rounds. Such a meeting may be a delicate experience for both professionals and patients since it moves established structures and manners in clinical work. The researchers convey how experiences of imbalance as well as of disorientation were displayed, both in relation to the professionals and patients. The study highlights the importance of interpersonal relationships in a situation often characterized by formality and tradition. The researchers conclude that the lifeworld approach clarifies the need for a reflected patient perspective in caring and for professionals to develop some kind of readiness to touch upon existential issues. Obviously, it is not enough for professionals to understand what patients say, but also to be aware of existential moods in the patient as well as in themselves. Such reasoning is valid also for social care and evaluators.

Another way to exercise one's expanded awareness is to benefit from the whole field of humanities and arts. In biographies, novels and other forms of fictive literature, there are many good descriptions of existential matters that include stories about illness, dysfunction, suffering, and dying as well as health, well-being, and how to manage one's life projects. Also film can contribute with lifeworld stories that illuminate existence and may activate a broader field of understanding than just reading is able to (Hörberg, Ozolins, & Ekebergh, 2011; Hörberg & Ozolins, 2012). The narrative power is immense. It illuminates existential meanings and add to the spectre of nuances in understanding life in a meaningful way for both care practitioners and evaluators, and may induce professionals with new ideas and develop new means of understanding someone or something.

In a study of patients' and clients' violence against professional carers it seemed that violence was experienced less likely to happen when patients were encountered in an undisguised and straightforward way, and when they sensed unrestricted respect (Carlsson, Dahlberg, Ekebergh, & Dahlberg, 2006). In these encounters the nonverbal communication was significant and not least was an *embodied moment* shown to be essential, a moment when not many words were uttered but still a full dialogue happened with facial expressions, glances, gestures and with presence. Professional carers who showed little interest, who were "hard faced" or never smiled, who did not notice or ignored the patients when they were upset, made them feel not understood and, moreover, to create a facade of indifference and "coldness" in themselves as well. The study concludes that having come to such a point, violence is close. The findings show persons longing for authentic care, the potential for nonverbal communication and a need for care professionals to improve this skill, in order to improve their capacity of understanding.

There is a whole field of *movement and contact improvisation* that can serve the need for expanded awareness and with which one can improve understanding and nonverbal communication. Even if verbal communication is included, the exercises mainly function by touching. Touch is an expressive form of contact, which has an immense impact on all living creatures. It can be experienced as an invitation or even a request that awaits some reply, as well as giving room for a sense of relief and permission to just be (Ozolins, 2011). Also Dahlberg and Gran (2015) point out the phenomenon as both threatening and pleasurable. They have presented an interesting idea of touch and describe ways to engage with others through *listening touch* (Dahlberg & Gran, 2015) in movement and contact improvisation. They emphasize the aim of putting oneself in play in a bodily dialogue that enacts questions such as: "Who are you?" and "Who am I?"

The nonverbal approaches probably find more reasonable use in care practice than in evaluation. However, I persist in addressing both care practitioners and evaluators, because even if all kinds of human relations, not least in evaluation, becomes transferred to verbal language, awareness of basic nonverbal communication is of immense importance. As I have shown above, human relationship has so many nuances, of which a great deal is wordless. Besides, there are lots of instances in health and social care where people do not have the ability to express themselves in straight words, for example children, persons with brain damage or dementia, or immigrants who lack the new country language skills. The awareness of how many facets our lifeworld has brings us to the claim of new epistemological approaches.

DEVELOPING NEW EPISTEMOLOGICAL APPROACHES

The idea of New Public Management (NPM) is central in the prevailing paradigm of health and social care. Modern health care has in a broad sense become an economically driven medical event, participating in a high-tech context associated with disease and to a large degree pharmacological treatment. As a consequence, all evaluation is governed by assumptions of what evidence is that allow only for methods which suits the prevailing paradigm. The ideal is Randomized Controlled Trials, where the outcomes are based on mathematics and statistics, an approach that suits hand in glove with medical drug treatment.

My experience from health care and research makes it obvious that very little in human existence is measurable; that even if mathematics is something exact, there is little in health care research that can benefit from the exactness. This is a fact that is too little debated. Even in social care we see similar effects of NPM such as a passion for measurements, and even here we see a widely spread use of diagnoses and other categorizations that reduce persons to something objective, measurable, and accountable.

I believe that there are many good and important aspects of modern care that are of importance, not least the development of cures of diseases that earlier was not available. However, we still face a situation where most health conditions that people seek care for are not curable. At the same time as we read about the most advanced surgery we can find many examples of people who try to overcome illness by their own, when health care cannot help them with their pain, experiences of being exhausted, or of being overwhelmed by meaninglessness. The technologization, categorization, medicalization, and econimization of health and health care have developed beyond any reasonable limits and what we now see is that health (and social) care, to a great extent, seems to have forgotten what it is all about. That illness is more complex than something a pill can cure. That health and social care is something that should engage people's existence and in particular how people's health and function in society play an essential part in their lives. That health and social care should deal with questions of well-being and how people can go through with the things they wish from life.

In research that relies on mathematics and statistics, called quantitative research, there must be a much more profound awareness of when and how this approach is valid. An outcome that is presented with nine decimals is not at all evident if the phenomenon of the research is not well defined and not defensibly measurable. Further, the mismatch between individualized care and statistics based on normal distribution must be problematized. Health and social care would further benefit from much more autonomous research that is based in language, called qualitative research, as well as mixed approaches including both quantitative and qualitative approaches. Also, qualitative research approaches need to be more advanced and to let go of studies that only mirror the current and general opinions or shallow beliefs, that just record what people say, instead of displaying the existential depths of people in illness or other forms of suffering. Unfortunately, also the shallow practise of qualitative research can be viewed as an effect of the positivist cover and based in the NPM paradigm, in research as well as in evaluations of care.

The NPM approach makes less good health and higher costs at the same time, because it is expensive not to consider the lifeworld of people, especially in the long run. And besides, NPM is not an ethical approach. I call for a development of new approaches of research and evaluation that match the real world of people, approaches that recognize the lifeworld.

LIFEWORLD-LED RESEARCH AND EVALUATION

Lifeworld-led research, research that is sensitive to the many facets of existential experiences, is of interest if we want to develop forms of practice and evaluation that are close to the web of life in patients and clients. We have already seen some above (cf. Ranheim & Dahlberg, 2012; Ekebergh, 2007, 2009, 2011; Berglund, 2014; Lindberg, Hörberg, Persson, & Ekebergh, 2013a, 2013b, 2015; Hörberg, Ozolins, & Ekebergh, 2011; Hörberg & Ozolins, 2012; Carlsson, Dahlberg, Ekebergh, & Dahlberg, 2006). These examples may function as role models for evaluation.

Lifeworld-led research gives room for lifeworld-led care, which gives patients, clients, and their lifeworlds "more voice" (Dahlberg, Dahlberg, & Nyström, 2008; Todres et al., 2014). Lifeworld-led research is more than, and in some ways different from, qualitative research. Although it can be seen as a form of qualitative research, lifeworld-led research is ontologically and epistemologically more solid than qualitative research in general, and its main aim is to go beyond the general level of opinion in favor of existential meaning (Dahlberg & Dahlberg, forthcoming; van Wijngaarden, van der Meide, & Dahlberg, 2017). Within a perspective of lifeworld-led research we search for knowledge of what health means to people in their everyday life, how illness and care involve with their deeper existential horizons, and how illness and care have impact on people's well-being and, not least, their capacity to manage their endeavors in daily situations. Understanding such lifeworld horizons goes beyond simple (descriptive and nonconclusive) case studies and accounts of people's experiences in their own words. The tradition of phenomenological research encourages a level of reflection and understanding in which both the shared and unique dimensions of people's experiences are communicated. It acknowledges that human experience is not just encompassed by local, private dimensions or by common, public ones (van Wijngaarden et al., 2017).

A lifeworld approach to research and evaluation is an open, insightful and pliable approach, where methods are chosen for the capacity to be receptive and susceptible enough to find and discover phenomena in focus. Such approach demands from the researcher to be attentive and open, and not making definite what is indefinite, that s/he does not stay in the everyday style that above is described as the natural attitude, which is characterized by fixed, almost closed, and especially un-problematized perspectives. With Cavalcante Schuback's (2006) words it is about adopting an attitude "that enables one to hold on to the patient meanwhile" (p. 139), thus being in that in-between, the movement between poles, where meanings come to be. Such an attitude may seem to be a simple task, but in our contemporary instant and quick-happening society, where multitasking is a necessity, it is far from simple. All investigators must exercise and practice the noble art of attentively dwelling, waiting for existence to show its many and deep meanings.

One important aspect of openness in investigations such as evaluations of care is to avoid ready-made political assumptions or to be driven by fixed theories. Without ignoring the economic problems that many nations have with their public sectors, I emphasize that it is the quality of health and social care that must be in focus, that is, that people find that due to the care they get, their health or social situation is better off, that the care meets with them where they are, in their everyday events, in their course of life.

For many years now, in most health care regions of Sweden, patients have been invited to fill in so called waiting room questionnaires, which show that patients are overall quite positive to the care. These surveys have been a main argument for not improving health care in many regions. Once I had the opportunity to interview one of the recipients of such a questionnaire. Sitting there in the waiting room, expecting to soon be asked in for a small but to him very important surgery, he was so very happy and grateful that finally, after months of waiting, he should be rid of the severe pain in the hip. So, having the questionnaire in his hand, he scored 9s on most questions, he told me. However, a few minutes after he had handed in the questionnaire he got the information that his surgeon had been called over to the emergency ward and that he would be asked in again in "only a few weeks." "If they had given me the questionnaire back I would have scored 2s over the whole line," he commented. When I asked him about his further experiences of health care he revealed much of anxiety, that he had not felt that the professionals listened to him and that he actually had no real power over his situation. He also revealed that there was no room in the questionnaire for such experiences.

Now, of course we cannot draw heavy conclusions from one interview, but it gives an interesting insight into the lifeworld and provides us with an example of how these kinds of surveys work in the human world. If they are NPM investigations disguised as quality of care evaluations, they are no good. It is not an act of evidence, and simply not ethical, to give questionnaires to persons, asking them to mark alternatives that do not adequately fit with their situation, that do not really address them and their experiences. This is instead a safe way to silence them. A better idea is to be clear about what purpose the evaluation has and then choose the right method to reach the goal.

THE NEED FOR PHILOSOPHY OF SCIENCE

According to my own experience from health care and research as well as from advising and reviewing in research, a main problem still is not that the majority of research is quantitative and that there is a lack of qualitative research. Instead there is a common bottom line for the problems in both quantitative and qualitative approaches, namely how even advanced researchers lack insights into philosophy of science, what scientific research really is about. It is however not surprising. In many European countries NPM, with its focus on transparency and cost control, goes hand in hand with a positivist approach to research which also spills over to the many uses of evaluations. In such practice the aim is already set and the main focus simply is upon method, how to practice a technique. The theory and presuppositions behind the methods that are in use are not being considered important. There is even, in many countries, neglect towards theory of science. In Sweden, as an example of the state of affairs, as well as in many similar countries, it is possible to earn a PhD degree without one single course on theory of science. This can be compared with engineers receiving their diplomas without any study of mathematics or physics.

For contemporary and coming challenges, we need better research and forms of evaluation than just practicing the method of measuring. We need awareness of how a range of scientific characteristics, such as ontological and epistemological foundations rule all kinds of methods and how they work, what phenomena they suit and what outcomes are possible. Without a sound insight into philosophy of science, the method is allowed to direct the whole investigation, instead of the more logic way around; that one chooses method after what phenomenon is in focus, what questions there are and what aim the study has. It is pretty much a simple task. In short: If the phenomenon of study is measurable, then we can utilize the full potential of mathematics and statistics. If the phenomenon belongs to the experiential domain, then verbal (including embodied) methods must be employed.

However, even here we run into grey zones and that is the proper place for mixed methods. Much more than today we should combine methods. For example, it would be advantageous to invite people to phenomenological interviews to explore the meanings that are involved when they score 1 or 10 or for that matter 5 in surveys. It would also be of interest to find out what characterizes the people (and their experiences) who we find in nonvalid signification zones. And vice versa, would it be of immense importance to use the outcomes of a phenomenological study to form a questionnaire that would give us a wider picture of some phenomenon.

In addition to what is already said it is important to emphasize that qualitative inquiry suffers from a similar problem as the quantitative, namely that the focus has been on following a method. Even within qualitative approaches there has been some kind of fear of philosophy. That is the only way to explain the frequent occurrence of "content analysis" in health and social care publications, in research as well as in evaluations. In this approach the interest is to simply record what people say about or what the opinion is of the care they have received, or something else. This lack of theory and deep analysis is fair enough if one wants to know if a person prefers green or red apples but if the focus is upon health, illness, life, and care, it is definitely not enough. Sometimes it is obvious that researchers have some kind of interest into this dilemma, when they add some experience, meaning, and interpretation to the methodological practice. However, since they avoid all kinds of scientific theoretical foundation they do not clarify what experience or meaning is or how it comes about, or what an operation such as interpretation demands from a researcher.

Even methods that sometimes are labelled *phenomenological, hermeneutic,* or *phenomenological hermeneutic* have to be inspected for their foundations. Sometimes we even in these instances can see how the step-by-step practice is pronounced more important than the insights into the epistemology that explicitly or implicitly guide the methodological movements. A consequence is that the references to methodological prescriptions often are shallow. These step-by-step approaches seem easy to follow and practice, not least for students, but even more experienced researchers or other investigators are attracted by the simplicity of these pragmatic approaches (Dahlberg & Dahlberg, forthcoming). Neither content analysis nor other step-by-step methods can serve evidence based interests (van Wijngaarden, van der Meide, & Dahlberg, 2017). There are too many weaknesses in these approaches.

CONCLUSIONS

In this chapter, I have explored understanding as a key phenomenon in health and social care practice as well as in all kinds of investigations of care. Both in care practice and care investigations such as evaluations of care, we need to understand the persons who are, have been or will be patients or other clients. My main argument is that in order to understand these people we must employ approaches that do not manipulate them by giving up living in them, but that—on the contrary—lead us to life, existence, and meaning. Both in care practice and in investigations of care, we must understand what and how the care does something to the person's life and health situation, how the care is experienced and received by the person and her/his environment, and if and how the care supports the person's plans and dreams for life. This is the profound meaning of care practice and inquiry and it is such understanding that can make health and social care effective in the word's most profound meaning. It is only when focus is upon the ethics of the lived world that we can talk about evidence in relation to health, caring and health care evaluation.

KEY CONCEPTS

- philosophy/theory of science
- phenomenology and hermeneutics
- lifeworld
- perception
- existential vulnerability
- qualitative methods
- quantitative methods
- mixed methods

DISCUSSION AND QUESTIONS

1. In the chapter there are some thoughts on how one knows that a person has understood. Reflect on how you generally see that understanding has happened. Reflect also on how you feel yourself when you sense that you have been understood.
2. Discuss verbal versus nonverbal communication, what are the similarities and differences, pros and cons?
3. What examples do you see of NPM in your everyday practice? How does this socioeconomic paradigm affect your daily life?
4. How can qualitative and quantitative methods be combined and what could the benefits be? What would be the difficulties?

NOTES

1. What also makes it a difficult trying to grasp Husserl's, is the fact that his texts were often handwritten or were lectures, which were edited by his assistants. Sometimes it is not easy to see which ideas are Husserl's original ones, and which have been completed by an assistant. There are examples of debates whether Husserl's philosophy should be interpreted in one or another way. When I have run into such questions in my reading and in the analysis that forms the central meaning of this chapter, I am mainly following the interpretation by Merleau-Ponty (cf. 1995, 2002, 2004) as well as Natanson (1973) and Elliston (1977). I am also avoiding such parts of Husserl's philosophy that belong to his most critiqued subjects (e.g., where he explicitly and intently works with concepts such as solipsism or egology).
2. I want to thank Shinji Hamauzu, Osaka University, for sharing his sincere insights into the Husserlian philosophy.

REFERENCES

Berglund, M. (2014). Learning turning points—in life with long-term illness—visualised with the help of the life-world philosophy. *International Journal Qualitative Studies on Health Well-being, 9,* 22842. Retrieved from http://dx.doi.org/10.3402/qhw.v9.22842

Carlsson, G., Dahlberg, K., Ekebergh, M., & Dahlberg, H. (2006). Patients longing for authentic personal care: A phenomenological study of violent encounters in psychiatric settings. *Mental Health Nursing, 27*(3), 287–305.

Cavalcante Schuback, M. (2006). The knowledge of attention. *International Journal of Qualitative Studies on Health and Well-being, 1*(3), 133–140

Dahlberg, H. (2013). *Vad är kött? Kroppen och människan i Merleau-Pontys filosofi* [What is flesh? The body and human being in Merleau-Ponty's philosophy]. Göteborg, Sweden: Glänta Produktion.

Dahlberg, H., & Dahlberg, K. (2003). To not make definite what is indefinite. A phenomenological analysis of perception and its epistemological consequences. *Journal of the Humanistic Psychologist, 31*(4), 34–50

Dahlberg, H., & Dahlberg, K. (2015). Vårdande mellanrum och sammanhang [In-between caring and its context]. In M. Arman, K. Dahlberg, & M. Ekebergh (Eds.), *Teoretiska grunder för vårdande* [Theory for caring practice], (pp.145–168). Stockholm, Sweden: Liber.

Dahlberg, H., & Grahn, E. (2015). Att skapa rum. Om beröring i rörselse. [Making room. On touching in movement]. In F. Sandström (Ed.), *Kroppsfunktion* [Body function]. Stockholm, Sweden: C.off.

Dahlberg, K. (2014). *Att undersöka hälsa och vårdande* [Investigating health and caring]. Stockholm, Sweden: Natur & Kultur.

Dahlberg, K., Dahlberg, H., & Nyström, M. (2008). *Reflective Lifeworld Research* (2nd ed.). Lund, Sweden: Studentlitteratur.

Dahlberg, K., & Dahlberg, H. (forthcoming). *Open and reflective lifeworld research—A third way.* Manuscript in preparation.

Dahlberg, K., & Ekebergh, M. (2015). En livsvärldsorieterad etik [Lifeworld-led ethics]. In M. Arman, K. Dahlberg, & M. Ekebergh (Eds.), *Teoretiska grunder för vårdande* [Theory for caring practice] (pp. 95–103). Stockholm, Sweden: Liber.

Dahlberg, K., & Segesten, K. (2010). *Hälsa och vårdande i teori och praxis* [Health and caring in theory and practice]. Stockholm, Sweden: Natur & Kultur.

Dahlberg, K., Todres, L., & Galvin, K. (2009). Lifeworld-led healthcare is more than patient-led care: An existential view of well-being. *Medicine, Health Care and Philosophy, 12,* 265–271.

Ekebergh, M. (2007). Lifeworld-based reflection and learning: A contribution to the reflective practice in nursing and nursing education. *Reflective Practice 8*(3), 331–343.

Ekebergh, M. (2009). Developing a didactic method that emphasizes lifeworld as a basis for learning. *Reflective Practice, Special Issue 10*(1), 51–63.

Ekebergh, M. (2011). A learning model for nursing students during clinical studies. *Nurse Education in Practice, 11,* 384–389.

Elliston, F. (1977). Husserl's phenomenology of empathy. In F. Elliston & P. McCormick (Eds.), *Husserl. Expositions and appraisals* (pp. 213–231). London, England: University of Notre Dame Press.

Gadamer, H.-G. (1976). *Philosophical hermeneutics* (D. Linge, Trans.). Berkeley: University of California Press.

Gadamer, H.-G. (1995/1960). *Truth and method.* Second revised edition (J. Weinsheimer & D. Marshall, Trans.). New York, NY: The Continuum.

Gadamer, H.-G. (1996/1993). *The enigma of health* (J. Gaiger & N. Walker, Trans.). Stanford, CA: Stanford University Press.

Halling, S. (2006). The emergence of the dialogal approach: Forgiving another (with Jan O. Rowe & Michael Leifer). In C. T. Fischer (Ed.), *Qualitative research methods for psychologists: Introduction through empirical studies* (pp.173–212). New York, NY: Academic Press.

Halling, S., & Leifer, M. (1991). The theory and practice of dialogal research. *Journal of Phenomenological Psychology, 22*(1), 1–15.

Heidegger, M. (1998/1927). *Being and time* (J. Macquarrie & E. Robinson, Trans.). Oxford, England: Blackwells.

Husserl, E. (1964/1928). *The phenomenology of internal time consciousness* (J. S. Churchill, Trans.). London, England: Indiana University Press.

Husserl, E. (1970a/1900). *Logical investigations: Vol. 1. Prolegomena to pure logic.* (J. Findlay, Trans.). London, England: Routledge & Kegan Paul.

Husserl, E. (1970b/1936). *The crisis of European sciences and transcendental phenomenology* (D. Carr, Trans.). Evanston, IL: Northwestern University Press.

Husserl, E. (1973/1948). *Experience and judgement* (J. S. Churchill & K Ameriks, Trans.). Evanston, IL: Northwestern University Press.

Husserl, E. (1977/1929). *Cartesian meditations* (D. Cairns, Trans.). The Hague, Netherlands: Martinus Nijhoff.

Husserl, E. (1998/1913). *Ideas pertaining to a pure phenomenology and to a phenomenological philosophy. First book* (F. Kersten, Trans.). London, England: Kluwer Academic.

Husserl, E. (2000/1928). *Ideas pertaining to a pure phenomenology and to a phenomenological philosophy. Second book* (R. Rojcewicz & A. Schuwer, Trans.). London, England: Kluwer Academic.

Hörberg, U., Ozolins, L-L., &. Ekebergh, M. (2011). Intertwining caring science, caring practice and caring education from a lifeworld perspective: Two contextual examples. *International Journal of Qualitative Studies on Health and Well-being, 6,* 10363. doi:10.3402/qhw.v6i4.10363

Hörberg, U., & Ozolins, L. (2012). Film as support for promoting reflection and learning in caring science. *Indo-Pacific Journal of Phenomenology, 12.* doi:10.2989/IPJP.2012.12.1.6.1114

Jingrot, M., & Rosberg, S. (2008). Gradual loss of homelikeness in exhaustion disorder. *Qualitative Health Research, 18*(11), 1511–23. doi: 10.1177/1049732308325536

Levinas, E. (1969). *Totality and infinity* (A. Lingis, Trans.). Pittsburgh, PA: Duquesne University Press.

Lindberg, E., Hörberg, U., Persson, E., & Ekebergh, M. (2013a). It made me feel human. A phenomenological study on older patients' experiences of participating in a team meeting. *International Journal of Qualitative Health and Well-being, 8,* 20714. doi:10.3402/qhw.v8i0.20714

Lindberg, E., Hörberg, U., Persson, E., & Ekebergh, M. (2013b). Older patients' participation in team meetings. A phenomenological study from the nurses' perspective. *International Journal of Qualitative Health and Well-being, 8,* 21908. doi:10.3402/qhw.v8i0.21908

Lindberg, E., Ekebergh, M., Persson, E., & Hörberg, U. (2015). The importance of existential dimensions in the context of the presence of older patients at team meetings. In the light of Heidegger and Merleau-Ponty's philosophy. *International Journal of Qualitative Study on Health and Well-being, 10,* 26590. Retrieved from http://dx.doi.org/10.3402/qhw.v10.26590

Merleau-Ponty, M. (1968/1948). *The visible and the invisible* (A. Lingis, Trans). Evanston, IL: Northwestern University Press.

Merleau-Ponty, M. (1987/1960). *Signs* (R. McCleary, Trans.). Evanston, IL: Northwestern University Press.

Merleau-Ponty, M. (1989a/1946/1947). The primacy of perception and its philosophical consequences. In *The primacy of perception* (J. Edie, Trans.). Evanston, IL: Northwestern University Press.

Merleau-Ponty, M. (1989b/1961). Eye and mind. In *The primacy of perception* (J. Edie, Trans.). Evanston, IL: Northwestern University Press.

Merleau-Ponty, M. (1991a/1964). *Consciousness and the acquisition of language* (H. Silverman, Trans.). Evanston, IL: Northwestern University Press.

Merleau-Ponty, M. (1991b/1969). *The prose of the world* (J. O'Neill, Trans.). Evanston, IL: Northwestern University Press.

Merleau-Ponty, M. (1995/1945). *Phenomenology of perception* (C. Smith, Trans.). London, England: Routledge.

Merleau-Ponty, M. (2002/1959–1960). Resumé of the course: Husserl at the limits of phenomenology. In L. Lawlor & B. Bergo (Eds.), *Husserl at the limits of phenomenology* (J. O'Neill & L. Lawlor, Trans.). Evanston, IL: Northwestern University Press.

Merleau-Ponty, M. (2004/1948). *The world of perception* (O. Davies, Trans.). London, England: Routledge.

Natansson, M. (1973). *Edmund Husserl. Philosopher of infinite tasks.* Evanston, IL: Northwestern University Press.

Ozolins, L. (2011). Beröringens fenomenologi i vårdsammanhang [The phenomenology of touch in caring contexts]. Linnaeus university dissertations, nr. 62.

Ranheim, A. (2011). *Expanding Caring—theory and practice intertwined in municipal elderly care.* Linköping University Medical Dissertation, No. 1217.

Ranheim, A., & Dahlberg, K. (2012). Expanded awareness as a way to meet the challenges in care that is economically driven and focused on Illness—A Nordic Perspective. *Aporia, 4*(4), 19–23.

Ranheim, A., Kärner, A., & Berterö, C. (2012). Caring theory and practice—Entering a simultaneous concept analysis. *Nursing Forum, 47*(2), 78–90.

Svenaeus, F. (2001). The phenomenology of health and illness. In K. Toombs (Ed.), *Handbook phenomenology and medicine.* Dordrecht, Netherlands: Kluwer Academics.

Todres, L., Galvin, K., & Dahlberg, K. (2014). "Caring for insiderness": Phenomenologically informed insights that can guide practice. *International Journal of Qualitative Studies on Health Well-being, 9*(1), 21421. doi:10.3402/qhw.v9.21421

van Wijngaarden, E., Leget, C., & Goossensen, A. (2015). Ready to give up on life: The lived experience of elderly people who feel life is completed and no longer worth living. *Social Science & Medicine, 138,* 257–264. Retrieved from http://www.sciencedirect.com/science/article/pii/S0277953615002889

van Wijngaarden, E., van der Meide, H., & Dahlberg, K. (2017). Researching health care as a meaningful practice: Toward a nondualistic view on evidence for qualitative research. *Qualitative Health Research, 27*(11), 1–10. doi:10.1177/1049732317711133

PART II

DEMOCRATIC EVALUATION FOR A CARING SOCIETY

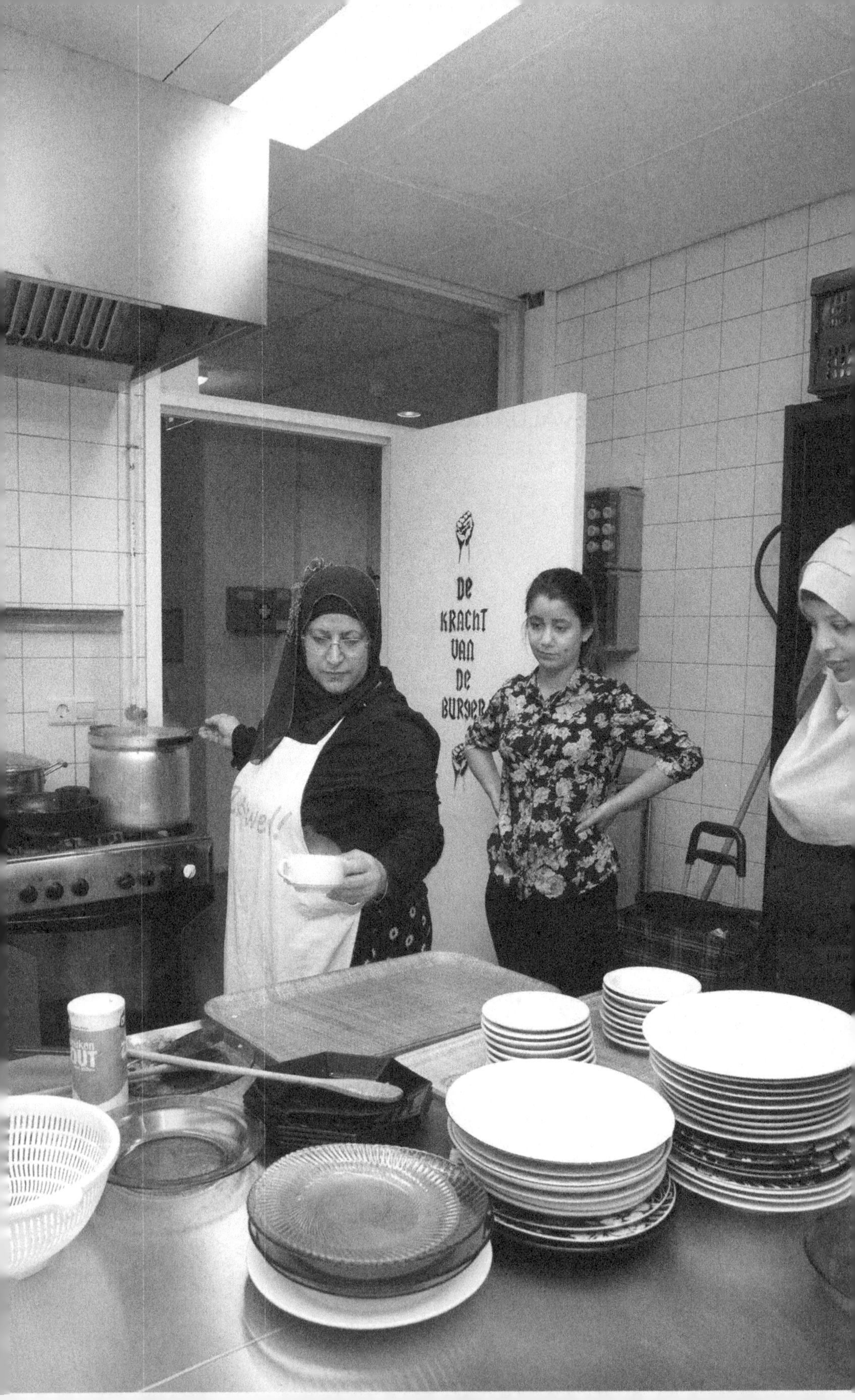
DE
KRACHT
VAN
DE
BURGER

CHAPTER 3

DEMOCRATIC EVALUATION AND CARE ETHICS

Helen Simons
University of Southampton

Jennifer C. Greene
University of Illinois, Urbana–Champaign

DEMOCRATIC EVALUATION

At the heart of democratic evaluation is the commitment to engage with and advance democratic values within the very process of the evaluation, making sure that all those with a legitimate interest in the evaluation have their perspectives heard and represented. Democratic evaluation strives also to ensure that beneficiaries and all citizens have access to the results of evaluations so they can contribute their own viewpoints and debate the issues at stake. This sounds reasonable and simple, but it is a complex process to enact. The process involves first the cultivation of multiple sets of relationships and second procedures that enable the honest gathering of data and safe sharing of perspectives, even if they differ. We return to this essential relational aspect of democratic evaluation in discussing how we practice democratic evaluation in the contemporary contexts in which we work. But first we outline the key premises and stances of democratic evaluation, and honor its origins and original authors.

Evaluation for a Caring Society, pages 83–102

Origins of Democratic Evaluation in the United Kingdom and the United States

Many approaches to evaluation can be said to be "democratically oriented" in that they aspire to influence the decision-making process by providing impartial, empirical evidence to help policy makers make informed decisions about policies, programs, and resources. However, this stance positions evaluation on the sidelines of democratic decision-making, giving over the power for dissemination and enactment of results to our elected public officials, thereby trusting them to do the right thing in the genuine public interest. Alas, too rarely do they do this right thing. And so evaluation that simply informs policy does not powerfully or consequentially advance democratic values or contribute to a democratic society. What is needed is a process of political engagement to ensure that evaluation is of consequence for those it affects and offers all citizens the opportunity to engage with and debate the findings.

Historically, there are two approaches that do engage directly with the political nature of evaluation by recognizing evaluation as "inherently and inevitably entangled with and constitutive of the politics and values of [public] decision-making" (Greene, 2006, p. 136). These are democratic evaluation as conceived by Barry MacDonald (1974) and deliberative democratic evaluation as advocated by Ernest House and Kenneth Howe (1999). In the processes advocated by these authors, democratic evaluation actually creates conditions for the discussion and interaction of the differing values and interests manifest in the context, implementation, and results of the evaluation. Our characterization of and commitment to democratic evaluation owes much to these authors, so it seems appropriate to describe briefly how each conceived the approach he advocates.

MacDonald's Democratic Evaluation in the United Kingdom

It was the early '70s in the United Kingdom when Barry MacDonald (1974, p. 17) first proposed a model of democratic evaluation. This was, in part, a reaction against technocratic models of evaluation. But most importantly, MacDonald's model acknowledged that all citizens—whatever their role in society—have the right to have their perspectives on important social issues recognized and the opportunity to discuss evaluation knowledge about these issues. This concept of democratic evaluation provides an alternative both to evaluation approaches that are dependent on the authority of the evaluator and the perceived rigor of methodology, and those that are circumscribed by the values and authority of the bureaucracy. Instead, it locates the process of conducting the evaluation in the ideals of a democratic society, in which access to knowledge and freedom of expression are core values. In incorporating different stakeholder interests and standpoints in the evaluation and making the evaluation process and results accessible to the wider public, MacDonald's (1974) democratic evaluation aspires to shift the power base and role of judgment in evaluation to a wider public constituency.

The central aspiration of MacDonald's (1974) democratic evaluation is to find a balance between a person's right to privacy and the public's right to know. It has three core concepts: *confidentiality, negotiation,* and *accessibility.* These concepts are translated into a set of ethical principles and procedures that provide a strategy for conducting the evaluation and ensure, through the negotiation principle, that the central aspiration is met. Confidentiality offers protection to those contributing to the evaluation that their privacy will not be invaded and that no un-negotiated data about them become public. Negotiation is the means to ensure that the data participants have offered as part of the evaluation are fair, accurate and relevant. Accessibility is guaranteed by the overriding principle of independence—of sponsors, programs, policies, and participants. Reports and findings are published, so that all citizens have the opportunity to consider and inform policy debate.

This principle of independence, in particular, is necessary, as in the United Kingdom there is a lingering tradition of secrecy or privacy in government and a legacy in the social system that encourages a certain deference. At the time the United Kingdom's democratic approach to evaluation evolved, openness and access to information were not as evident as they were (and still are) in the United States. It was not automatic that all evaluations became public. This may help to explain both the choice of the key concepts—confidentiality, negotiation, and accessibility—and their interrelationships, even interdependence. In particular, negotiation was considered central to ensuring that evaluations became public and that the citizenry was indeed informed about them.

House's Deliberative Democratic Evaluation in the United States

For almost as long as Barry MacDonald, Ernest House has championed a democratic approach to evaluation. House's American version of democratic evaluation seeks primarily to address inequities of social class and minority culture and to advance social justice in both the contexts at hand and in the broader society (House, 1990, 1993; House & Howe, 1999). House attends specifically to the ways in which evaluation not just influences but actually serves to constitute public decision-making institutions and discourses, and thereby policy directions.

In collaboration with philosopher colleague Kenneth Howe, House developed a *deliberative democratic* model for evaluation (House & Howe, 1999, 2000). This model intentionally ensures that the *interests* of all stakeholders, specifically those of the powerless and the poor, are respectfully and consequentially included. The model rests on three interrelated principles:

1. *Inclusion of the interests of all legitimate stakeholders.*
2. *Dialogue*—A process through which the *authentic interests* of diverse stakeholders are identified.
3. *Deliberation*—The rational process by which varying, even conflicting, stakeholder claims regarding the evaluand are negotiated. Deliberation is a form of reasoned discussion, with evidence and argument.

Deliberative democratic evaluation is a challenging ideal to implement because existing arrangements of power and privilege render equitable, authentic participation by all stakeholders difficult to actualize. But, of course, the very point of this theory is to conduct evaluations that help to redistribute power and privilege in more just and equitable ways.

There are many similarities between democratic evaluation and deliberative democratic evaluation in terms of the inclusion of all invested interests and values; the importance of dialogue, negotiation, and deliberation; and the challenging nature of evaluation's role in political and policy contexts. In both traditions, it is up to the evaluator to ensure (to the greatest extent possible) that all perspectives are indeed represented, and that conditions are established that facilitate equitable opportunities to dialogue and debate so that extant power structures do not dominate. MacDonald is more prescriptive than House in specifying precise procedures to help ensure such equitable access and deliberation. House leaves it more open for each evaluator to find the most appropriate approach, but insists on inclusion, dialogue, and deliberation as core values and thus elements in the process.

In a recent paper (Simons & Greene, 2014) we speculated on how the background of these two authors led to their strong commitment to democratic values and to the specific model each generated. That is not our precise purpose in this paper. Nevertheless, we wish the reader to keep in mind, in considering what follows that, just as with the two authors mentioned above, our *own* values and biographies, along with the particular sociopolitical tenor of the times in which we have lived and worked, influence which evaluation models we espouse. They do not stand alone.

Democratic Evaluation: Our Theory and Practice

Our views on democratic evaluation are anchored in the premise that *all* evaluations advance some values and that we need to explicitly state and take responsibility for which values are promoted in our work. Our views are further centered in our belief that democratic values are the most defensible ones we can advance in our practice—methodologically, politically, socially, and ethically. The key principles in our vision are these. Democratic evaluation:

- Explicitly advances core values of equity, access, justice, fairness, and human dignity.
- Is inclusive of the values and interests of *all* legitimate stakeholders.
- Negotiates the generation of evaluation knowledge through procedures that are equitable, fair and just.
- Is independent of vested or powerful interests in the management structure for the evaluation, in the evaluation process, and in reporting.
- Is educative in the process of conducting the evaluation and in providing robust, fair-minded evaluative knowledge to inform ongoing public debates about important social issues.
- Is accessible (in language, content, and form) to policy makers, practitioners, beneficiaries, and citizens, so that all can contribute to the policy making processes of our societies.
- Is of consequence, that is, it makes a difference to people's lives, especially those who experience disadvantage.
- Is ethical in respecting the human dignity of all individuals with regard to their concerns and differences.

These principles are translated into a set of procedures to guide the conduct of the evaluation, and ensure the principles are enacted in practice. Examples are:

- All participants will be granted equal opportunity to contribute to the generation of evaluation knowledge.
- Evaluation reports will be negotiated with those concerned on criteria of accuracy, relevance, and fairness.
- No one person or group will have the right to veto the external evaluation report (Simons, 2010).

With procedures such as these, as Norris (2014) has recently stated, "Democratic evaluation tries to create the social conditions for organizational and institutional learning. It is a strategy for enabling a democratic society to live up to its ideals and aspirations" (p. 5).

These principles and procedures, and the values that underpin them, encapsulate our aspirations for democratic evaluation. Our enactments of these aspirations may fall short, at times, of reaching their full potential. Shortfalls can and do inevitably occur—for reasons beyond the remit of the specific evaluation, such as economic constraints, competing political agendas, and practical limits on the evaluator's influence and power. Yet they are vital aspirations to maintain, even in straitened times. As we said in the opening to this section, all evaluation is steered by some set of principles, procedures, and values, for which the evaluator must assume responsibility. We assume this responsibility through our beliefs that democratic evaluation offers a strong counterpoint to the performative and economically-driven public discourse so dominant today and so highly controlled by the top one percent. Democratic evaluation creates possibilities for all citizens to have the worth and authority of their perspective acknowledged *and* to have a voice in public decision making.

EXPLORING THE CARING DIMENSIONS OF DEMOCRATIC EVALUATION

In this section we indicate how we adopt a caring perspective in our work as democratic evaluators. In a subsequent section, we examine how selected key concepts of care ethicists may relate to our work.

It is clear in the account above of our perspective that we strongly endorse an ethic of caring in our practice as democratic evaluators. In this section, we argue that as democratic evaluators we adopt an ethic of caring in our work in two principal ways. First, we deliberately establish caring relationships in our professional evaluation practice as consonant with the democratic principles of human dignity, fairness, and inclusion. Second, our views of democratic evaluation are anchored in our commitments to epistemic justice, itself a principle of care and caring. These two caring anchors of democratic evaluation are elaborated next.

The Central Role of Relationships in Democratic Evaluation

We take the view that establishing and nurturing the right relationships with evaluation stakeholders[1]—from commissioning, designing, and conducting the evaluation to reporting the findings—is essential to creating the conditions for the effective generation of honest, defensible evaluation knowledge that is inclusive of diverse interests and values in the evaluation context. This goes beyond the customary respectful (and "caring") ways in which many evaluators socially and politically interact with stakeholders, ways that instrumentally help us to establish credentials, gain access and stakeholder buy in, and gather valid and useful data. Most importantly, these relationships are necessary for creating evaluation spaces and places for inclusive dialogue, with and among diverse stakeholders. Such places afford *all* those with a legitimate interest in the evaluation, irrespective of power and position, the opportunity to discuss the meanings and implications of the evaluation findings and to have their perspectives and experiences heard and validated. In other words, it is in the relational fabric of evaluation that democratic commitments to fairness, equity of voice, and epistemic justice are enacted and safeguarded.

Shifting for a moment to our voice as zealous advocates for democratic evaluation:

> It can never be a question of whose side the evaluator is on. It can never be a question of colluding with the most powerful of stakeholders. It can never be a question of excluding marginalized stakeholders just because it is logistically difficult to include their experiences and viewpoints. It can never be a question of caving in when an evaluation report is criticized or attempts are made to censor it. There are always multiple perspectives to be heard and represented. And it is indeed a fine-tuned juggling act to maintain faith with all stakeholders while favoring none, to negotiate the inclusion of different values, and to attend to legitimately different interests. Democratic evaluation is a practical political art. Not for the fainthearted. Nor reliant on simply producing a methodologically sound report. Such a report is a clear evaluative responsibility but cannot, in and of itself, advance the values of democracy.

In short, it is through the cultivation of respectful and inclusive relationships at all levels that not only are the values of democratic evaluations advanced, but also the conditions laid for the uptake of any implications from the evaluation for policy decision-making and action.

A Commitment to Epistemic Justice

The second fundamental parameter of our democratic evaluation practice is our commitment to epistemic justice. This construct offers a vital philosophical justification for democratic evaluation, in addition to those frequently advanced, such as the politics of choice (MacPherson, 1965) and the egalitarian premises of John Rawls' (1971) theory of justice. The concept of epistemic justice defines truth as arising from the knowledge and experiences of *all* who are involved in a given set of social interactions, especially from those who are marginalized in the system (Fricker, 2007). Following feminist epistemologies, epistemic justice is "premised on the idea that perspectives drawn from the margins of any given discourse are not only different from mainstream perspectives, but [their inclusion] results in more truthful representations of the world" (Frank, 2013, p. 364). This, of course, is an epistemological and ethical, as well as a political, point. Evaluations that do not engage with the truths of all involved in the evaluation, at whatever level in the formal structure they are, will fail to determine the truth status of the program. In practice what this means is that we have to work harder at the relational level to establish trust, to uncover the meanings of the less articulate or those who fear possible consequences of speaking out, and to resist the pressures of those who wish to fob us off. The origins for this argument are briefly presented below.

Origins of the Concept of Epistemic Justice

The concept of epistemic justice arose from critiques of the radical relativism of *epistemic diversity*, a critique to which those of us who hold a relativist position on social knowledge may wish to listen particularly well. Epistemic diversity posits that diverse paradigms (including traditional post-positivism, social constructivism, feminisms, post-structuralisms, and so on) *each start from a different set of assumptions about the social world*, so there is no way to adjudicate among them. Hence we are left with, "What is true for you is true for you" and "What is true for me is true for me" (Frank, 2013, pp. 363–364).

What is needed, therefore, is a rejection of the radical relativism of epistemic diversity in favor of a strong commitment to inclusion and equity of voice. This is precisely what democratic evaluators have been advocating for decades; the concept of epistemic justice makes the argument at the philosophical level. This concept further encourages those with power in the social world as currently configured to take more seriously the diversity of voices in our evaluations.

> If the perspectives of those positioned without power in our social world go unheard, then our collective epistemic resources are less robust than they otherwise would be. This situation is one of "epistemic injustice." Those without power are silenced and this leads to an incomplete and inaccurate [understanding] of the social world. (Frank, 2013, p. 365)

Here is the thought in different words.

> We silence large segments of the community of knowers, of which we are all a part, at our own peril. The truth of our social world will elude us until we learn what it means to *hear* [emphasis added] across the social spectrum. (Frank, 2013, p. 365)

Reprise: On "Care" and "Caring" in Democratic Evaluation

Here we summarize our argument so far.

- Democratic evaluators are attentive to the ethics and politics of care in their practice, fully cognizant of the multiple interests that inhabit that context.

- Democratic evaluators engage in caring relationships in their work in multifarious ways throughout the evaluation. It is through genuine and respectful relationships with all stakeholders that our commitment to democratic values of equity, fairness, and epistemic justice is realized.
- Our commitment to epistemic justice, in particular, sculpts our commitments to radical inclusion of voice, experience, and standpoint. This demands that the defensible generation and valuing of knowledge about a particular context or situation *must* include all the "knowers" in that context.
- Our democratic understanding of the "politics of care" invokes questions like: "Are all important stakeholders represented in this conversation?," "Do all have opportunities to join the conversation?," "Do we need an interpreter for any key stakeholder groups?," "How shall we organize the seating in the room so all places are on the same level and none appears privileged?," and "How shall we moderate an evaluation situation where the most powerful stakeholders dominate and seek to diminish the perspectives of those less powerful, either through dismissal or censorship?"

Example: Caring in a Multi-level Complex Evaluation

Here is an example of how one of us (Helen) adopted a caring ethic in a democratic evaluation she aspired to conduct in a country different from her own ("aspired" because the context in which it took place was unfamiliar culturally and hierarchical relationships were the norm). Two different features of this evaluation evoked and challenged a caring response from the evaluator, the first interpersonal and the second administrative and political.

The project was funded by the European Union with a remit to train novice evaluators in evaluation methodology and processes, while they were conducting a case study evaluation of an educational transformation in their country. The European Union funding for the program was located in a government department and was managed both by a person in that department and an advisor from abroad, creating two levels of program oversight. It was a difficult political context in which to train evaluators. The leaders of the evaluator trainees were senior in their academic disciplines but did not have experience in evaluation, their mother tongue was not English, and they were not accustomed to working in groups, as required by the structure of the training (teams of four) and evaluation work in the field. So, care had to be taken at the beginning of this project to establish caseworker–trainee trust in the English evaluators doing the training, as well as trust amongst the trainees themselves, to support functional collaboration within and across evaluation teams. Caring for each person in the team was also important to ensure that his/her contributions were valued, given the customary deference to the authority structure in the culture in which the trainees lived and worked.

Caring shifted to an administrative and political level when the final report was challenged by the in-country manager of the program. This manager's challenge was deep and wide, even to the point of trying to insist that blame (for program limitations or shortcomings noted in the case reports) be attributed to certain people and that excerpts from interviews be modified or omitted to put specific other people and the program in a more positive light. Negotiations ensued for several months. Meanwhile, the funding for the program, including the pay for the case study evaluators, was held up. The final report had to be formally approved before the case evaluators received the money due to them for work already completed.

In this context the democratic evaluator had to honor the work conducted and had to care for the integrity of the evaluation, for the financial well-being of those who carried out the evaluation, *and* for the manager, even though he was holding the evaluation to ransom unless changes were made. I (Helen) understood that in this culture, the manager may have feared for his job if he endorsed a report that, in his perception, did not present his country in a favorable light. Yet, I also understood that in that context I was the guardian of the evaluation that the case evaluators had conducted, of the promised pay for their work, and of the risks to their well-being and livelihoods if payment was not forthcoming. I was also aware that eventually the project had to report on the use of funds to the European Union. The challenge was how to care for all in a complex, multi-level political context, while trying to resolve an impasse and ensure that the core responsibility of the evaluator to present a defensible public evaluation report was upheld.

There were three ways in which I aspired to balance these conflicting needs. The first was to speak personally with the manager and the leaders of the evaluation teams to try and understand what their personal fears were and from where they stemmed. For the manager, it was mostly about the next job; for the case evaluators, it was about commitments they had made to their families and, as senior academics, to the academic rigor of their work. Each had a legitimate worry and a position to uphold. The second was persuasion—to engage the different key actors in this context to empathize with the "other" and to understand that some compromise would be needed on all sides. The third was reason—to negotiate what was reasonable in that context to resolve the situation. It was not surprising to find that the personal took precedence in people's minds over the other two strategies of persuasion and reason. Trying to balance care for individuals and their needs at the same time as caring for the validity and legitimacy of the project, which was not without impact on the standing of all involved, was stressful and extended well beyond the original terms of reference. I could have taken a different route and reported directly to the European Union. That would have resolved the payment issue for the case evaluators but not kept faith with the management protocols of the project. So I desisted and managed the project stress while endeavoring to reach at least a satisfactory outcome for all involved.

PARALLELS AND TENSIONS BETWEEN DEMOCRATIC EVALUATION AND CARE ETHICS

In this section, we first share our preliminary understandings of core ideas in the care ethics literature in the context of the health (and human service) professions, and second consider how these may or may not be congruent with the values and aspirations of democratic evaluation. We raise possible differences as *tensions* in order to respectfully explore the possible connections between these two domains of practice. The literature we draw on is selective. We focus on writings that offer some resonance with our work as democratic evaluators. The primary sources on which we draw are Abma and Widdershaven (2008), Hankivsky (2014), Hamington (2014), Noddings (1984), Tronto (1993, 2010), and Van Heijst (2012).

To start, we briefly consider how care is defined by some of these writers, as these definitions suggest a potential difference between our role as evaluators and how those who adopt a care ethic in the health professions see their role. In early conceptions, caring was viewed as a moral action in relation to another human being (Noddings, 1984; Tronto, 1993; Lindeman, 2005). One cares for or about someone, often someone who is in a state of stress or suffering, and often someone for whom the carer has the responsibility to safeguard that person's welfare. This conception of care ethics is underscored by the following definition of the field. "Care ethics, as an interdisciplinary field of study, regards people to be dependent upon one another for their survival, development, and social functioning, and highlights the unchosen obligations we all have towards others by virtue of our interdependency" (Engster, 2007, p. 7).

More recently the concept of care is being considered beyond the interpersonal to address the political and institutional structures of care (Hamington, 2014; Tronto, 1993, 2010). Tronto (1993, 2010), in particular, has argued that as care is a practice fundamental to our social life, it has to be considered in a political context, not simply as a private or professional moral relationship between two individuals (Lindeman, 2005, p. 97).

It will be readily apparent even from this brief description of the concept of care that there are differences in purpose, role, and practice between democratic evaluation and caring in a health context. In the first place, the major purpose and responsibility of evaluation is not to care per se, but to deliver an evidential base for decision-making regarding a social program or policy. Secondly, evaluators are not subject to institutional customs and norms of caring. Whatever "caring" we practice in our evaluations is voluntary and nonbinding. We are not asked to take responsibility for any one individual's welfare. And thirdly, our role is usually temporary; we have no institutional commitment to "care" beyond the term of the evaluation.

Let us hold these as temporary differences while we explore further key ideas about care from a care ethicist's perspective.

Conceptualizing Care From Care Ethicist's Perspective

We present in this section several themes and ideas we observed in our review of selected literature on care ethics.

Care is an Inter-Relational Moral Activity

A number of care theorists (e.g., Noddings, 1984; Lindeman, 2005) discuss care as an interrelational responsibility of one individual for another, even while they question the social and political implications of such a conceptualization. Given that many caring practices are carried out by women and others who are marginalized and are often not well paid, care bounded by this remit can potentially aggravate extant inequities, for both the carer and the person cared for. This is not always the case, of course, but it is a danger.

Care is a Sociopolitical Construct

Other theorists (see, for instance, Tronto, 2010; Held, 2006) view care as a public social issue, rather than just a private responsibility that is typically shouldered by women. These scholars argue that care is a sociopolitical construct, not simply a construct that describes some of our relationships with one another. In particular, central to Joan Tronto's (2010) provocative conceptualization of care are claims that care is more than moral ethics and more than a relational social practice; it is also normative and political (p. 160). Thus, she argues, the problems that should be addressed by care are problems of "purpose, power, and particularity" (p. 161). This crosses the boundary between politics and personal morality as Hamington (2014, p. 200) points out. With the introduction of this broader political purpose we can begin to see a possible connection to democratic evaluation, which we maintain is how evaluation in the public sphere *should* be conducted.

Care is the Integration of an Empathetic Process and a Political Responsibility

In this conception, care is constructed as having two faces, for each of three different characteristics.

- First, care can cross the boundary between an imaginative and emotional process of empathy and one's political responsibility as a citizen. That is,

  > caring is an imaginative process that engages empathy... and therefore the act of care has political potential because we can imagine caring for others in similar ways or imagine others caring for one another in similar ways. [Caring becomes] experiential knowledge imaginatively extended to others with implications for political change. (Hamington, 2014, p. 200)

- Second, because care has this emotional component and is anchored in relationships with others, caring can cross boundaries *between relational and epistemic knowing.* "Emotion provides the requisite motivation to learn more about the unknown and distant others as well as to act on their behalf" (Hamington, 2014, p. 210).
- Third as a political construct, care crosses the boundaries between private and public life. It erases the boundary between the relegation of care and caring to the private sphere and the assumption of public, societal responsibilities for the provision of care. It thus becomes part of inclusive conversations and debates about public priorities and responsibilities and raises the potential for actually valuing the practice of care and for redressing the inequities in care provision and practice in societies around the world.

This recognition of the multiple countenances of care in context resonates with the relational and political intent in our evaluations, our emphasis on epistemic justice in democratic evaluation, and our strong intention to influence policy debate on social issues.

Care is Integral to a Strong Democracy

Many care theorists explicitly conceptualize a care ethic as integral to a strong and sustainable democracy. Notably, Engster and Hamington (2015) maintain that the theory of care is related to the development of both self and citizenship. And Tronto (2010) argues that caring practices and institutions in a genuine democracy should attend to three inherent dimensions of care: power, particularity, and purpose. Further, "the practice of care describes the qualities necessary for democratic citizens to live together well in a pluralistic society, [and thus] the implications for moral education are enormous. Only in a just, pluralistic, democratic society can care flourish" (p. 206).

In an earlier paper, Engster (2004) critiques extant conceptual arguments by care theorists on the particular connections between care and democracy, and then offers his own "institutional caring political theory." Engster's democratic perspective on care and caring has three categories of rights: (a) rights related to development and dependency work, for example, child care; (b) political and economic rights, for example, rights to freedom of speech, religion, assembly, press; protections from arbitrary or cruel and unusual punishment; as well as rights to bodily health and economic sustenance; and (c) rights to equitable political participation by all. In other words, paraphrasing Engster, a caring democratic society requires the development of caring institutions.

Clearly, these views of care—as a public good that is fundamental for a strong democracy—are consonant with our own commitments to democratic evaluation. Enacting a democratic and caring approach to evaluation is a further challenge.

Tensions in the Practice of Care Ethics Within Democratic Evaluation

The *responsive evaluation practice* that is articulated by the editors (and some authors) of this volume is an example of how a democratic ethic of care can be incorporated, even fully integrated, into evaluations of caring practices. Building on the original responsive evaluation work by Robert Stake (1983), Tineke Abma, Merel Visse, and Guy Widdershoven—along with their colleagues and students—have constructed a form of responsive evaluation that focuses on the political dimensions of caring practices (Abma, 2006; Abma & Widdershovern, 2008, 2011; Visse, Abma, & Widdershoven, 2015). This Dutch-born form of responsive evaluation intentionally engages the plurality of human care experiences and interests, alongside the inequalities and power asymmetries that infuse care contexts. Many of these care contexts concern health and physical–emotional well-being. Commenting on the political aspect of their conceptualization, these authors note that:

> Care is more than a virtue, bound to persons. Ontologically, care ethics as a political ethics is grounded in a relational paradigm that honors interdependence in caring relationships and the constant changes in positions of vulnerability and fragility. People are seen as interdependent, meaning: "[A]ll humans are vulnerable and not vulnerable at different points in their lives." (Visse, Abma, & Widdershoven, 2015, p. 167)

At first sight this may appear similar to how we engage with the political and power differentials in democratic evaluation. However, interdependence in caring relationships as described above is beyond the remit of our evaluation task *where the program or policy is not explicitly a caring practice.* As democratic evaluators we attend seriously to how we purposefully engage fairly and compassionately, with diverse stakeholders and thereby demonstrate caring for all in our evaluations. But caring is not an explicit responsibility of our craft. And extant power differentials among stakeholders are engaged in our practice through explicit procedures designed not around caring, but rather to promote equity of voice in the generation of evaluative knowledge and to advance epistemic justice.

Nevertheless, in what follows we have tried to address two questions: "How could a view of care, as advocated by the care ethicists we consulted, practically contribute to our work as democratic evaluators?" and, conversely, "How might our democratic evaluation practices, intrinsically political in any event, connect to the practice of care espoused by care theorists and practitioners?" These challenging questions are taken up in a set of four tensions we believe are likely to surface as we engage the implications of care ethics for our practice.

Attaining Fairness and Equity

The democratic evaluator must act fairly and be perceived as fair, rather than partial, by multiple diverse stakeholders. To be fair, the democratic evaluator may need to make special efforts to reach or hear from particular stakeholders, namely, those with least power and voice, including the intended beneficiaries of the program being evaluated. These special efforts are motivated by a concern for epistemic justice, which is catalyzed by a valuing of equity.

The work of an evaluator from a care ethicist's perspective would likely be more personal, enacted through a stance of conveying actual caring to particular individuals or groups in a given evaluation context, identified as the opportunity or need for caring arises.

These different guiding frameworks for action could be in tension with one another. For example, do I keep my painstakingly-arranged appointment with a program participant, aiming to hear her experiences and viewpoints of the program, or do I respond to the staff member in front of me who is expressing some distress about his multiple program responsibilities? Or how do I do both, without unduly upsetting the context and extending the time frame of the evaluation?

Criteria for Judging Program Quality

The democratic evaluator judges program quality using democratic criteria of equity, justice, and fairness. A good program is one that advances these democratic ideals in ways that matter concretely and sustainably for intended program beneficiaries and others with an important stake in the program. More specifically, the democratic evaluator is concerned about the equity, justice, and fairness of program *access, participation,* and *outcomes.* Do all eligible program participants have equal opportunities to sign up for and actively join the program? Do all have equally positive program experiences, and do all have equally strong program outcomes? "Equally" here does not mean the same quantitatively but rather, in qualitative terms, having comparable importance in one's life.

The evaluator who takes a care ethicist's perspective for evaluating a health or well-being program judges program quality using criteria expressive of care and being cared for. A good program is a caring program, one in which participants feel deeply and genuinely care for and cared about. And this caring is important in ways sustainable for participants' well-being.

These different criteria are not inherently in conflict. Still, imagine an evaluation context in which data on a range of program outcomes indicate that the fewest targeted benefits accrued to those most in need. That is, the program functioned to increase inequities in targeted outcomes, and so would be judged a failure by a democratic evaluator. Yet, in interviews, participants from this "most in need" group reported that they felt well cared for in the program—findings that could inspire the evaluator from the caring professions to judge the program a success.

Whose Truth and How to Reach It?

As indicated earlier, the democratic evaluator adheres to a concept of epistemic justice, which means the results of an evaluation are only true if they fairly represent the views of those at the margins or those difficult to understand, beyond the views of the more articulate, powerful, and visible.

The "caring" evaluator, according to some care ethicists, takes the view that truth emerges through care. For example, Thayer-Bacon (2000) says "connected knowing is based upon an epistemology that emphasizes truth as something that emerges through care" (p. 79).

There is a possible tension here regarding which version of the truth (both equally legitimate) should prevail. The democratic evaluator's inclusive and balanced analysis of the program's strengths and weaknesses? Or the report from the care ethicist's perspective, demonstrating that the program events, while intending to support participants through emotionally-difficult times, were not experienced as safe, supportive or caring?

"Every Realm of Life"

The democratic evaluator evaluates a particular program or policy. This may be in health, education, social welfare, or some other field. But, it is a particular, circumscribed set of activities and intended outcomes, and the responsibility of the democratic evaluator is to report fairly, justly, and equitably on that program.

The "caring" evaluator, according to some care ethicists, focuses on care in particular situations (Leget, van Nistelrooij, & Visse, 2017), on understanding what good care is, both within and outside health care settings, including, for example, care for the environment or for cultural heritage.

These are different boundaries for our respective work that could be complementary and mutually enhancing. Or they could invoke tensions and frictions between commitments to democratic equity and commitments to the ethics of care.

REPRISE AND REFLECTION

Democratic evaluators attend closely to the relational dimensions of their work, because equity of voice for all relevant stakeholders is fundamental to defensible evaluation practice *and* because it is through these relationships that democratic ideals are realized, or not. Care professionals attend closely to the relationships established in their work, because that *is* their work—caring is fundamentally integral to meaningful human relationships and to ensuring that people are cared for and get well. People who feel genuinely cared for will recover from illness more quickly or experience significant improvements in their quality of life. Some democratic evaluators privilege care and caring as central to all democratic practices. And some care ethicists attend to the fairness and justice embodied in relationships, as constitutive of the norms and values of the broader society. So, professionals in both fields attend closely to the relational fabric of the contexts in which they work, and to the democratic ideals germane to these contexts—equity, justice, fairness—even as our work contributes to different societal and professional purposes and aspirations.

What we have considered in this paper is what more we could learn from each other. We have examined, for instance, how realistic it would be to judge program quality by the extent to which the program demonstrated deliberate and effective attention to caring in its implementation and intended and realized outcomes. This would be an unusual addition to the normal ways in which program quality is judged in our profession, which may not find favor with our colleagues or be seen as relevant by commissioners in government-sponsored evaluations. It may also be hard to accomplish, given the time scale and temporary nature of our evaluations.

Looking at the issue from a care ethicist's perspective, we wonder how incorporating democratic ideals of equity and justice as essential dimensions of a "good" caring context might influence the effectiveness of caring practice and the social and political aspirations of the field of care. At a policy level, we can see a possible resonance in the reconstruction of care ethics as a political construct, as care ethicists and practitioners seek to influence policy contexts (through arguing for more resources, higher pay for carers, better working conditions, etc.). These actions parallel the work of democratic evaluators as we democratize our findings in order to influence the policy debate to pay attention to epistemic justice and to accord more resources to programs of demonstrable democratic worth.

These suggestions need further deliberation. We raise them here as points of resonance, while acknowledging that the differences in our role and responsibilities are likely to lead to different decisions and practices in our respective fields. For there are certain parameters of our fields that require different codes of practice and that have different consequences for people in our respective professions.

KEY CONCEPTS

- democratic evaluation
- epistemic justice
- fairness, justice, and equity
- primacy of relationships

DISCUSSION QUESTIONS

1. The authors argue that democratic evaluators judge program quality on the fundamental democratic criteria of equity and justice. In what ways could the addition of a quality criterion of "caring" complement and even enhance these democratic criteria, toward a more fulsome and powerful evaluation?
2. The authors propose an ideal of *epistemic justice,* which defines truth as arising from the knowledge and experiences of *all* who are involved in the program/contexts being evaluated, especially those on the margins. How is epistemic justice related to caring?
3. How might the tensions raised by the authors of this paper be resolved to enhance both democratic evaluation and care practices in the health professions?

NOTE

1. In democratic evaluation, legitimate stakeholders are defined as all those with an interest in the program. This includes those with resource authority over

the program (policymakers, funders); those with administrative and implementation responsibility for the program (program administrators, staff, and volunteers); and intended participants in or beneficiaries of the program, their families, and their communities.

REFERENCES

Abma, T. A. (2006). The practice and politics of responsive evaluation. *American Journal of Evaluation, 27*(1), 31–43.

Abma, T. A., & Widdershoven, G. A. M. (2008). Evaluation as social relation. *Evaluation, 14*(2), 209–225.

Abma, T. A., & Widdershoven, G. A. M. (2011). Evaluation as a relationally responsive practice. In N. K. Denzin & Y. S. Lincoln (Eds.), *The Sage Handbook of Qualitative Research* (pp. 669–680). Thousand Oaks, CA: SAGE.

Engster, D. (2004). Care Ethics and Natural Law Theory: Toward an Institutional Political Theory of Caring. *Journal of Politics, 66,* 113–135.

Engster, D. (2007). *The heart of justice: Care ethics and political theory.* Oxford, England: Oxford University Press.

Engster, D., & Hamington, M. (2015). *Care ethics and political theory.* Oxford, England: Oxford University Press.

Frank, J. (2013). Mitigating against epistemic injustice in educational research. *Educational Researcher, 40*(7), 363–370.

Fricker, M. (2007). *Epistemic injustice: Power and the ethics of knowing.* New York, NY: Oxford University Press.

Greene, J. C. (2006). Evaluation, democracy and social change. In I. F. Shaw, J. C. Greene, & M. M. Mark (Eds.), *The Sage Handbook of Evaluation* (pp. 118–140). London, England: SAGE.

Hamington, M. (2014). Care as personal, political, and performative. In G. Olthuis, H. Kohlen, & J. Heier (Eds.), *Moral boundaries redrawn: The significance of Joan Tronto's argument for professional ethics, political theory and care practice* (pp. 195–212). Leuven, Belgium: Peeters.

Hamington, M. (2015). Politics is not a game: The radical potential of care. In D. Engster & M. Hamington (Eds.), *Care ethics and political theory* (pp. 272–292). New York, NY: Oxford University Press.

Hankivsky, E. (2014). Rethinking care ethics: On the promise and potential of an intersectional analysis. *American Political Science Review, 108*(2), 252–264.

Held, V. (2006). *The ethics of care: Personal, political, and global.* Oxford, England: Oxford University Press.

House, E. R. (1990). Methodology and justice. In K. A. Sirotnik (Ed.), Evaluation and Social Justice: Issues in Public Education. *New Directions for Program Evaluation, 45,* 23–36. San Francisco, CA: Jossey-Bass. Eric Number; EJ407899

House, E. R. (1993). *Professional evaluation: Social impact and political consequences.* Newbury Park, CA: SAGE.

House, E. R., & Howe, K. R. (1999). *Values in evaluation and social research.* Thousand Oaks, CA: SAGE.

House, E. R., & Howe, K. R. (2000). Deliberative democratic evaluation. *New Directions for Evaluation, 2000,* 3–12. doi:10.1002/ev.1157

Leget, C., van Nistelrooij, I., & Visse, M. (2017). Beyond demarcation: Care ethics as an interdisciplinary field of inquiry. *Nursing Ethics,* doi:10.1177/0969733017707008

Lindeman, H. (2005). Feminist ethics of care and responsibility. In H. Lindeman (Ed.), *An invitation to feminist ethics* (pp. 85–104). New York, NY: McGraw-Hill.

MacDonald, B. (1974). Evaluation and the control of education. In B. MacDonald & R. Walker (Eds.), *SAFARI 1: Innovation, evaluation, research and the problem of control* (pp. 9–22). Norwich, England: Centre of Applied Research in Education, University of East Anglia.

MacPherson, C. B. (1965). *The real world of democracy.* Oxford, England: Oxford University Press.

Noddings, N. (1984). *Caring. A feminine approach to ethics and moral education.* Berkeley, CA: University of California Press.

Norris, N. (2014, April 9). *Barry MacDonald and the democratic tradition in evaluation: Some lessons for the future.* Keynote address, UK Evaluation Society Annual Conference, London, England.

Rawls, J. (1971). *A theory of justice.* Cambridge, MA: Harvard University Press.

Simons, H. (2010, April). *Democratic evaluation: Theory and practice.* Paper prepared for the Virtual Conference on Methodology in Programme Evaluation. University of the Witwatersrand, Johannesburg: Wits Programme Evaluation Group. Retrieved from http://wpeg.wits.ac.za/main_site/downloads.htm.

Simons, H., & Greene, J. C. (2014, October). *Against the Odds but worth it: The value of democratic evaluation in contemporary society.* Keynote address at the European Evaluation Society, Dublin, Ireland.

Stake, R. E. (1983). Program evaluation, particularly responsive evaluation. In G. F. Madaus, M. Seriven, & D. L. Stufflebeam (Eds.), *Viewpoints on education and human services evaluation* (pp. 287–310). Boston, MA: Kluwer-Nijhoff.

Thayer-Bacon, B. J. (2000). *Transforming critical thinking: Thinking constructively.* New York, NY: Teachers College Press.

Tronto, J. C. (1993). *Moral boundaries. A political argument for an ethic of care.* New York, NY: Routledge.

Tronto, J. C. (2010). Creating caring institutions: Politics, plurality and purpose. *Ethics & Social Welfare, 4*(2), 158–171.

Van Heijst, A. (2012). *Professional loving care.* Leuven, Belgium: Peeters.

Visse, M. A., Abma, T. A., & Widdershoven, G. A. M. (2015). Practising political care ethics: Can responsive evaluation foster democratic care? *Ethics & Social Welfare, (9)*2, 164–182.

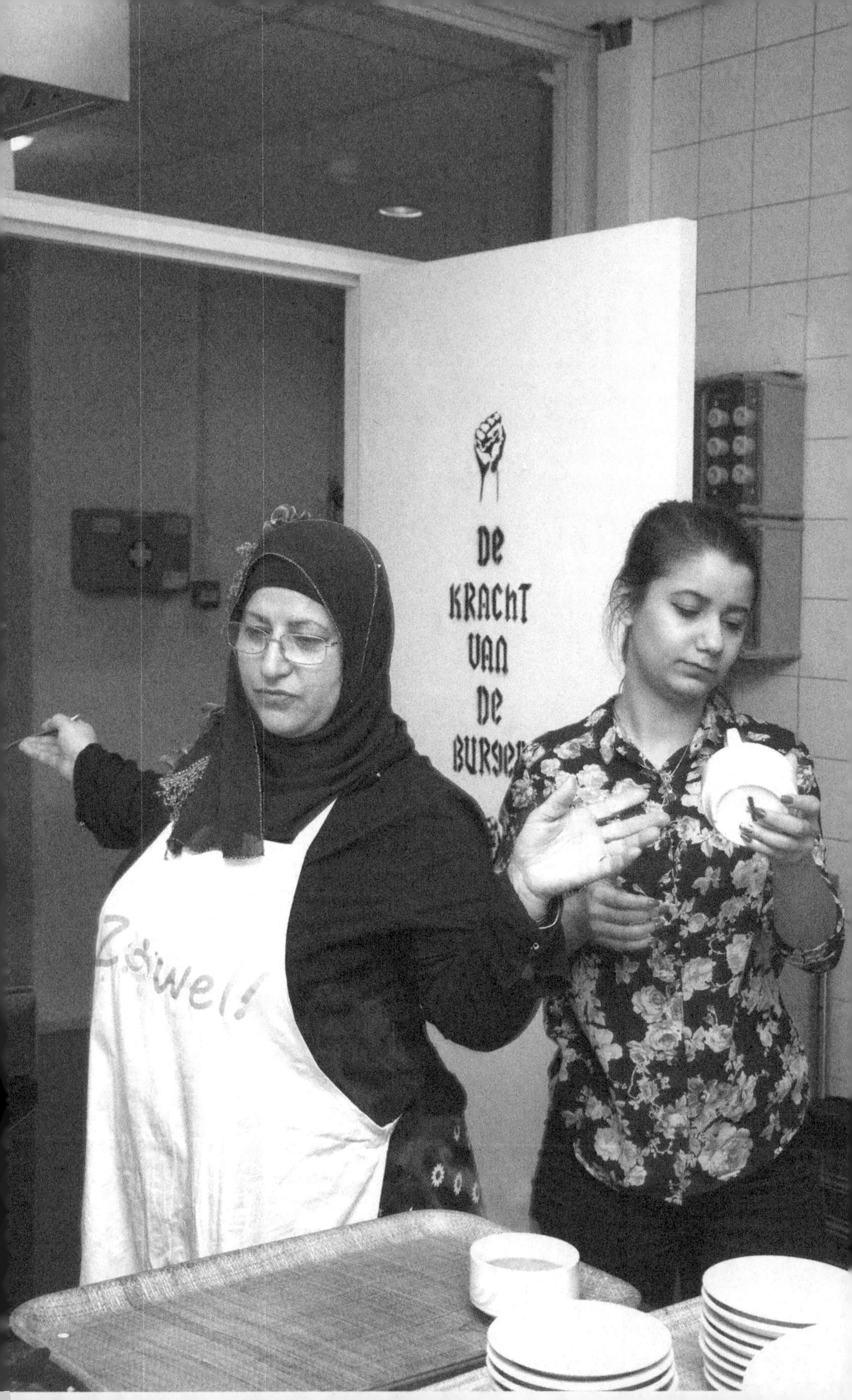
DE
KRACHT
VAN
DE

CHAPTER 4

DEMOCRATIC CARING EVALUATION FOR REFUGEE CHILDREN IN SWEDEN

Anders Hanberger
Umeå University

What is a democratic caring (DC) evaluator and what does it mean to be one, especially in terms of practicing responsibility for the stakeholders one works with in evaluation contexts? This chapter discusses the challenging issue of the responsibilities of evaluators, citing an evaluation of the reception of unaccompanied and separated children (UASC) in Umeå, a northern-Swedish community of over 100,000 residents. DC evaluation does not refer to a new evaluation approach. The notions of DC evaluation and the DC evaluator are used here in discussing what it means to be an evaluator who develops evaluation within a democratic and caring society. The discussion builds on both democratic evaluation and care theory. It is suggested that an enlightened DC evaluator is informed both by democratic evaluation and by research into good care, applying this knowledge reflectively during the evaluation process. This chapter discusses what is involved in

Evaluation for a Caring Society, pages 105–124

developing a DC evaluation with a special focus on the evaluator's responsibilities and good care.

The chapter continues with a brief presentation of the case: a democratic evaluation of care for a group of refugee children in Sweden. Subsequently, the theoretical underpinnings of democratic evaluation are presented. The next section discusses what DC awareness means and the responsibilities of a DC evaluator, illustrating this with examples from the case. The chapter concludes by considering what DC evaluation implies for the good care of refugee children.

THE CASE: DEMOCRATIC EVALUATION OF CARE FOR A VULNERABLE GROUP OF REFUGEE CHILDREN

UASC constitute a particularly vulnerable group of refugees. Since 2006, when the United Nations High Commissioner for Refugees (UNHCR) started collecting statistics on them, such refugees have increased steadily in numbers (UNHCR, 2014). In 2012, more than 20,000 asylum applications were filed by UASC (UNHCR, 2012). Two-thirds of these UASC applications were received in Europe; about 3,600 of these were received in Sweden, making the country the largest European recipient of UASC asylum applications per capita (UNHCR, 2012).

An unaccompanied child who arrives in Sweden and applies for asylum is first offered a temporary place to stay and then assigned to a municipality. The social services in that municipality, in this case Umeå, are responsible for the child's care and are required to investigate and assess the child's needs and to find suitable accommodation. Caring for UASC involves a variety of professional caregivers, such as social workers, care home staff, legal guardians, teachers, and other school staff, including school nurses. For example, coaches or mentors at care homes are responsible for creating safe homes, establishing everyday routines, providing children with information about Swedish society, helping them adapt to their new environment, stimulating them to become active, and supporting their efforts to learn Swedish. Each municipality also appoints a legal guardian and ensures that all children for which it is responsible are enrolled in education as soon as possible.

The municipality of Umeå signed an agreement with the Swedish Migration Board stipulating that Umeå should provide accommodations for at least 40 UASC per year. In early 2013, there were two municipal care homes and one supportive housing facility in Umeå. There was also an additional care home run by a voluntary association, the YMCA. The supportive housing comprised several apartments in which UASC lived in pairs, preparing themselves to live in apartments on their own and finally leave the reception system by the time they become 21 years old.

Unaccompanied refugee children have often experienced violence and war, dangerous journeys to host countries, impoverished living conditions in refugee camps, and sometimes abuse. Research into UASC reflects different assumptions about this group's vulnerability and needs. One stream of research into UASC concentrates on the children's vulnerabilities, psychological health problems, and human rights (cf. Derluyn & Broekaert, 2007; Fazel & Stein, 2002; Fekete, 2007; Shamseldin, 2012). These studies reveal that UASC are more likely to suffer from severe symptoms of anxiety, depression, and post-traumatic stress than are children accompanied by parents or relatives (Derluyn & Broekaert, 2007). In contrast, other studies emphasize the resilience and strengths of children, and demonstrate that UASC resettle, endure, and cope well, provided they are safe, are surrounded by supportive and trustworthy people, can maintain relationships with family and relatives, and are given an opportunity to educate themselves and live everyday lives characterized by predictable routines (Carlson, Cacciatore, & Klimek, 2012; Kohli, 2011). Taken together, research into and evaluation of UASC reception have identified factors crucial for successful reception and integration. These include

> stable and secure living conditions, access to social networks and social capital to maintain relationships with family and friends, supportive people and links to the majority population, access to education, predictable everyday routines, the quality of reception (i.e., commitment and competence of caregivers), and successful inter-organizational cooperation among service delivery actors. (Hanberger, Wimelius, Ghazinour, Isaksson, & Eriksson, 2016)

To support and evaluate the reception of unaccompanied refugee children in Sweden, the author of this chapter, together with four co-researchers, conducted a democratic evaluation of the reception of UASC in Umeå in 2012–2013 (Eriksson, Ghazinour, Hanberger, Isaksson, & Wimelius, 2014). The project was co-financed by the European Refugee Fund and Umeå University. The purpose of the evaluation was to: describe and analyze the reception system for UACS in Umeå, 2012–2013; draw conclusions on the achievement of objectives and on effects and consequences; and provide recommendations for improving care for the children. The democratic evaluation considered four components: problem situation, local reception system, implementation, and consequences (Hanberger, 2001a). The *problem situation* was broken down into the context, background, stakeholders, key actors, and various perspectives on the reception of unaccompanied children. The *local reception system* was described and the relevant program theory (i.e., how the intended effects were assumed to be achieved) was reconstructed. The analysis of *implementation* focused on the organization of reception in practice and the implemented measures. Cooperation between the children's caregivers, documentation, and individual and collective actions were described and assessed. The assessment of *consequences* concentrated on results, achievement of objectives, and consequences of the reception system for UASC and key actors. In addition, we identified and interpreted the values and features of the reception system that were promoted and reinforced from various perspectives (i.e., the multicultural, governance, interorganizational cooperation, and resilience perspectives). The evaluation of the reception program reflected the key stakeholders' views and experiences. Finally, we presented a progress report and a final report at several dialogue meetings.

VIGNETTE: DEMOCRATIC EVALUATION OF CARE FOR UASC

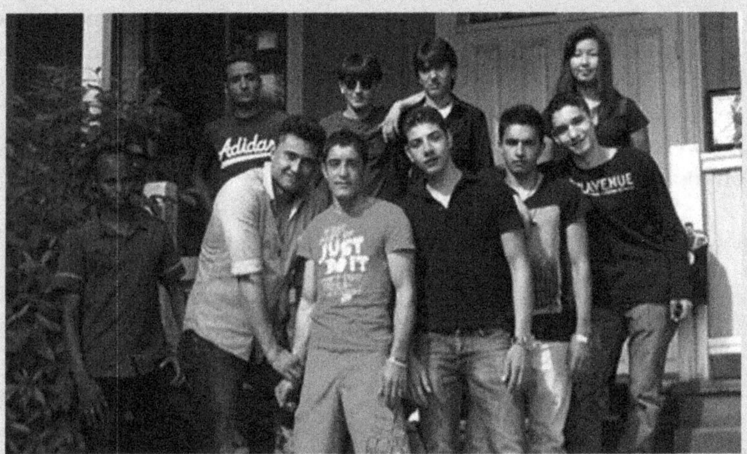

Photo 4.1 A group of UASC gathering in front of their care home in Umeå, Sweden.

In the everyday practices of supporting the refugee children, it soon becomes clear that some caregivers perceive the children as vulnerable, traumatized, and in need of psychiatric care, dependents for whom society should provide extensive care. Other caregivers adopt a more skeptical attitude toward UASC, for example, suggesting that the children get too many services and support, which tends to make them spoiled: "We create small request machines of these young people." Still other caregivers consider them strong, resilient individuals, and as potential resources to society. In this view, the challenge is how to support the UASC to become responsible adults: "You have to understand and explain that they are children who need support and coaching, not treatment and care." It is a difficult balancing act to help them manage various situations, according to some caregivers. The balancing act is expressed in terms of alternating between "walking first and showing the way," "walking beside and supporting," and "walking a step behind to let them try for themselves." It is important that the support be based on the children's needs and initiatives.

That these differences in perceptions of the children partly reflect the orientations in the literature became clear when evaluating the UASC program. During the evaluation process, we, the evaluators, interacted with key stakeholders in various ways. For example, we discussed how to formulate questions about the children's experience of care homes at a dialogue meeting with care home staff. According to the legal rules and reception policy, refugee children should be involved in choosing their care homes. If the children are actively involved in and can influence major decisions about their future, their wellbeing and integration will be facilitated. Therefore, among other things, we wanted to ask them: "Do you know why you are staying at this home?" and "Do you know that you are staying here voluntarily?" Care home staff questioned this approach, however, because such questions could affect the children's well-being and satisfaction with their care home.

> Yes, they should be informed about why they are staying here, but this is primarily a task for the social worker. We receive the children and work hard to make them feel at home, but if you give them the impression that they can move to another home, this can affect their willingness to adapt and can create restlessness.

In response to this concern, we decided to change our evaluative question to: "Have you been informed about why you are staying here?" and "Have you been informed that you are staying here voluntarily?" These small changes were important to the staff, helping them trust the evaluation and boosting its legitimacy. We did not discuss this issue with the children because the staff thought that this would create undesirable stress in them.

The vignette illustrates different attitudes toward the children and their needs among caregivers. Although the children are in a relatively weak position, being without their families, waiting for asylum decisions, and not speaking Swedish, some staff maintained that not all unaccompanied minors were necessarily traumatized and in need of special and extensive care (Eriksson, Ghazinour, Hanberger, Isaksson, & Wimelius, 2013).

The vignette also illustrates matters that evaluators need to be aware of, such as creating preconditions for trust and acknowledging multiple views. Besides the fact that UASC constitute a group of individuals who are perceived in different ways, views of what constitutes good care for these children vary within and among caregiver groups (e.g., social workers and care home staff). The vignette also illustrates that the evaluator needs to be responsive to multiple issues and concerns at the same time, including the legal rules of the reception system, the different roles of caregivers, and experiences of what affects UASC well-being and adaptation. Evaluators can therefore expect to encounter varied experiences and views of the reception system when interacting with UASC and various caregivers. Furthermore, an evaluator who cares for the children's well-being and integration must also be responsive to policy makers' and the general public's knowledge needs and provide accounts that can be used to support policy improvement and accountability. Before I elaborate on this matter, I first describe the theoretical and methodological underpinnings of democratic evaluation.

THEORETICAL CONSIDERATIONS

Democratic Evaluation

I have identified three approaches to democratic evaluation based on democratic theory, approaches that will be used to inform the discussion in this chapter (Hanberger, 2006).

Elitist democratic evaluation (EDE), the first approach, is based on elitist democratic theory (Schumpeter, 1942). The main role of EDE is to serve the decision makers' information and knowledge needs and provide feedback to enhance learning and accountability. On behalf of citizens, the decision makers (i.e., the elite) want to know whether or not an intervention has worked and its goals have been achieved. Different elites (i.e., political and/or administrative elites) can be supported, informed, and gain or lose support as a result of an EDE (cf. Farazmand, 1999a, 1999b).

Participatory democratic evaluation (PDE), the second approach, is based on participatory democratic theory (Pateman, 1970) and assumptions of self-governance. The main functions of PDE, as this approach is understood here (cf. Hanberger, 2006), are self-learning, empowerment, and self-determination. PDE concentrates on whether the participating and affected citizens or clients are included in and empowered by the policy or program, as well as throughout the evaluation process. The evaluation is designed by the clients/citizens themselves with assistance from an evaluator whose role is to facilitate and coach self-reflection and empowerment. In a sense, the evaluator acts as a coach for self-determination. The evaluation pays attention to preconditions and incremental progress made in the program or according to the client's own agenda.

Discursive democratic evaluation (DDE), the third approach, is based on deliberative or discursive democratic theory (Dryzek, 1996, 2000; Gutmann & Thompson, 2004; Habermas, 1996; House & Howe, 1999) and reflects House and Howe's (1999) deliberative democratic approach. DDE is primarily intended for collective learning (i.e., to meet the main stakeholders' practical knowledge needs) in order to justify collective action and facilitate public debates that enhance collective learning. The assumption is that local knowledge or time- and context-bounded knowledge could help participants and democratic society to further social improvement. DDE seeks to involve all legitimate stakeholders, citizens in particular, in the evaluation process and to assess the program according to criteria considered relevant by all legitimate stakeholders. The evaluator acts as a mediator and counselor by bringing arguments and analysis into the learning processes. The general public benefits from such evaluations through their production of accessible information and insights that help ordinary citizens become better informed about the performance of policies and programs, and through their facilitation of citizen participation in public debate. The DDE orientation has been developed as a "dialogical strand of responsive evaluation" (Abma, Leyerzapf, & Landeweer, 2016) that pays attention to power asymmetries in care practices and balances the needs of "the system world and life world" through dialogue (Abma, Leyerzapf, & Landeweer, 2016, p. 2; cf. Visse, Abma, & Widdershoven, 2015).

Responsibilities of Evaluators

The evaluator's responsibility to the stakeholders differs somewhat between the three models. An EDE evaluator adopts the expert role and has the responsibility to give the public access to results and to inform them of the misuse of evaluation if needed. In contrast, a PDE evaluator would have the responsibility to support and speak *for* the people being assisted, adopting the role of advocate, facilitator, and coach. These roles are intended to support self-governance in the ways indicated above. A DDE evaluator has the responsibility to give the public access to results and to inform them of the misuse of arguments and evaluations. The main role of the DDE evaluator, however, is to act as a mediator and counselor, with the special task of including *weak* and neglected perspectives and seriously considering various arguments and power asymmetries (Abma, Leyerzapf, & Landeweer, 2016). Furthermore, the mediating role includes creating mutually respectful processes and striving to build consensus through argumentation. It is disputable whether it is possible to promote the interests of the weakest through DDE and whether it should be the evaluator's role to strive to build consensus (Abma, Leyerzapf, & Landeweer, 2016; Hanberger, 2006; House & Howe, 1999; Picciotto, 2015).

Although the roles of a democratic evaluator vary depending on the notion of democracy applied, the three democratic orientations imply responsibilities for democracy and citizens that, for example, a technocratic

(Hanberger, 2001b) or bureaucratic (MacDonald, 1976) evaluation does not assume.

Responsibilities for Good Care

Care researchers draw attention to the fact that care is a multidimensional concept and that good care involves caring for, caring about, and responsiveness to the needs of the care-receiver as well as taking account of the responsibility of the caregiver (Tronto, 1993). Tronto (2014a) claims that good care includes a moral dimension linked to these notions of care, as well as a responsibility to foster good relationships and trust between the caregiver and care-receiver. Others emphasize the interdependence between people and that all are vulnerable. Tronto (2014a, 2014b), for example, points out that everyone is a care-receiver and caregiver at certain times of life. Widdershoven and Huijer (2001), who compare Nussbaum's Aristotelian ethics with the ethics of care as a social practice, demonstrate that these two ethical approaches conceive the fragility of care and one's responsibility for care in different ways. An Aristotelian approach draws attention to the fragility of care and the fact that caregiving involves choosing between conflicting values. One should be aware of one's own endeavors, take responsibility for one's choices, and respect values that one cannot endorse. It is important to adjust and reconsider care if it does not work as expected, and then be open to new ways of dealing with the situation. In contrast, an ethics of care as a social practice puts more emphasis on the fact that care entails sustaining life by engaging with others in joint practices. In this approach, the fragility of care is also experienced in its failures. Dealing with the fragility of care calls for openness to needs that have not yet been met. Care practices can only be corrected based on responsiveness to and communication with all parties involved, according to the latter approach.

What is conceived as *good* quality in care has also been defined in relation to the structural attributes of the care setting (e.g., indicated by staff competence), the processes of care, how care is performed (e.g., indicated by continuity), and the outcomes of care (e.g., indicated by the achievement of national care objectives; Donabedian, 1988/1997). Continuity, often measured as process or outcome quality, is also central to fostering a sound relationship between caregiver and care-receiver (Ingvad, 2003; Noddings, 1984; Szebehely & Trydgård, 2012; Wærness, 1984). Jerak-Zuiderent (2015) claims that the quality of concrete care and accountable care cannot be separated: good and accountable care is conceived as situated in the concrete situations of concrete people, meaning that care and accountability are intertwined.

When we connect notions of care with democratic evaluation, we may ask what theory of good care implies for a democratic caring evaluator. In addition to caring, a DC evaluator also needs to be aware of safety and security issues. Good care implies that measures are taken to prevent threats and violence and that routines are developed to manage them if they occur. The evaluator should be aware, for example, that disappointed asylum seekers who receive negative decisions on their asylum applications or receive negative news about family members can become frustrated and act without control. Caregivers and the evaluator need to be aware of this, act sensitively, and take safety precautions.

A caring evaluator, informed by research into good care, reflects on care-receivers' varying needs as a group and as individuals. He or she accounts for different caregivers' notions of good care, pays attention to issues deemed important by research into good care, and considers whether important aspects of care are being overlooked.

DEMOCRATIC CARING AWARENESS IN EVALUATION OF RECEPTION OF REFUGEE CHILDREN

This section applies the cited research and evaluation experiences to reflect on what DC awareness can imply in evaluating the local reception of refugee children.

How the Refugee Children Were Perceived

The above vignette illustrates three conceptions of the refugee children. These conceptions and attitudes interact with how problems and challenges are perceived by different stakeholders. If the children are conceived as traumatized and in need of psychiatric care to heal past wounds and integrate in a new country, the challenge is to treat them as fragile and provide individual care to satisfy their specific and changing needs. In contrast, if UASC are conceived as strong, resilient people, the challenge is to support and encourage them in line with growing expectations. If they are conceived as spoiled, the problem is understood as a cut-down problem: UASC should, for their own good, be offered less care and fewer services, and be taught to take more responsibility. All these approaches, but in particular the first and last, risk becoming protective care. Tronto (2016) makes a useful distinction between protective and democratic care, and the children are perceived differently if caring is conceived from a protective or democratic care perspective. Protective care fits into a hierarchical framework in which certain highly placed people protect from aggression those assigned to their care as weak and vulnerable. Protective care is informed by what Tronto calls masculine values, and may lead to resistance among children. Noncooperation can occur when care-receivers are not satisfied with the care they receive. We hear the fear of provoking this kind of response among some caregivers.

Democratic caring, on the other hand, is a joint and intersubjective activity (Widdershoven & Huijer, 2001). Tronto (2016) elaborates: "What caring democracy equalizes, then, are not acts of caregiving, but responsibilities for care—and as a prerequisite, the discussions about how those responsibilities are being allocated... *and assuring that everyone can participate in those allocations of care as completely as possible*" (p. 6). This joint decision-making about caring responsibilities fits better with the focus on the children's resilience, because this balances power asymmetries. Democratic caring also includes responsiveness, which means adjusting care when it is not received well and is evoking resistance responses. Democratic caring also entails a willingness to reflect on interactions that may cause recalcitrance. Democratic caring was recognized when caregivers deliberated on how to manage various challenges and joint responsibilities in networks set up for UASC (Hanberger et al., 2016).

Perceptions of (Good) Care

UASC have varied beliefs and values that can create conflicts between themselves and other children and between themselves and care home staff. For example, conflicts can arise during meals regarding what one should or should not eat. As discussed, such conflicts can be grounded in hierarchy and power asymmetry, and might be induced by interactions with and the paternalistic and over-protective attitudes of staff, all of which call for reflection. Tensions can also emerge because of, for example, growing frustration while awaiting an asylum decision or lack of privacy at the care home. The vulnerability of children can evoke an aggressive response among caregivers, which is then met by recalcitrance (Tronto, 2016). Cultural clashes can occur in schools due to the different values held by UASC and ethnic Swedes. Attention should be paid to the children's values while being aware of cultural differences, including the values and norms of the majority society, an issue to which I will return later.

An observation in the evaluation was that caregiver groups perceived their own care as "good care," whereas other caregivers were perceived as providing lower-quality care. A difference became evident between perceived good care and good reception in terms of the accommodations provided to the children. The public accommodations consisted of different types of housing services, each staffed with different types of personnel. In contrast, the YMCA's care home was more integrated. The same staff group and mentors followed the children even when they moved to external apartments. Most interviewed caregivers perceived the latter arrangement to work better, because of better continuity.

The children themselves were pleased with most of the reception spaces, with a few exceptions. A lack of natural places for meeting Swedish youths and obstacles to getting in touch with them, including staff integration measures, were perceived as problems. Staff engagement, empathy, care, encouragement, and practical support were valued by the UASC, who conceived these qualities as constituting good and genuine care. The children also emphasized that caregivers should have the right education and experience to provide good care and support. This resonates with Tronto's virtues of good care, namely, attentiveness, responsibility, and competence. Tronto (2014a, 2014b) points out that good care is more than simply a moral attitude, but is also hard, laborious work. This is precisely what the children noted, that care was not only paying attention and listening, but also offering practical support. Among those children who had already left the reception system, the caregivers who were the most engaged were the most appreciated. They noted that different types of caregivers (e.g., care home mentors, legal guardians, school teachers/staff, and social workers) treated them differently, though this was not described as problematic.

The local government and the Social and Welfare Committee responsible for implementing diversity policy and for organizing and coordinating the reception within and across municipal boundaries and civil society did not describe what they consider good care except as it is reflected in official goals. These goals reflect a legal responsibility approach to care and the notion of protective care: That is, good care occurs when UASC are provided the same conditions as all children living in the community, including protection of their rights and security.

Threats or violence were not evident in our material and most of the children felt safe and secure in their care homes. At the time the evaluation was conducted, the number of UASC was small. Today safety and security routines have become much more important due to the increased number of UASC, and due to events such as burnings of accommodations or schools and the killing of a staff member of a UASC housing facility in southern Sweden. A reception system based on the notion of protective care (Tronto, 2016) has consequences for how UASC are perceived and how care is developed for the children. UASC may act with resistance or apathy if they are not engaged in adapting care to their needs or are not expected to contribute to society.

Caregivers' Roles and Responsibilities

Social services are responsible for the child's care and are legally required to investigate and assess the child's needs and to find a suitable care home.

They also develop care plans and implementation plans to meet each child's needs and must follow up on implementation plans. Although it is their responsibility, it was impossible for them to follow up each child because of lack of time. Demands in the system world, according to Habermas (1996), restrict communicative action and, according to Abma, Leyerzapf, & Landeweer (2016) prevent the taking of moral responsibility.

The right to a legal guardian, a layperson who voluntarily works with the UASC to safeguard the child's interests until he or she becomes 18 years old, is regulated in Swedish law. The legal guardian is also responsible for managing the child's finances and other assistance. Depending on individual needs, circumstances, and ambitions, the legal guardians have more or less contact with UASC, care home staff, and schools. This reflects different understandings of the legal guardian's role and engagement. Although their prescribed role is to protect the children's interests, the evaluation found that some legal guardians did little to protect their interests, failing to provide good care.

Schools also have important responsibilities in UASC reception. Each Swedish municipality is responsible for enrolling children in education as soon as possible after their arrival. Most of those assigned to Umeå first took a 6-week introductory course at an upper secondary school. Most children continued on to an upper secondary school program emphasizing the Swedish language. Teachers and school nurses were also involved in supporting the children and were perceived as important figures in their lives.

The caregivers adopted different roles and responsibilities, and interpreted their mandates differently, which influenced what they did and how they discharged their responsibilities. In terms of Tronto's two approaches to care, a protective care approach clearly dominated, though some caregivers took on a broader moral responsibility reflecting a DC approach.

Caregivers' Collective Responsibility

UASC reception is a shared responsibility involving a wide range of actors, from the social services and county councils to civil society. Successful reception requires inter-organizational cooperation that promotes the gradual independence and integration of UASC in the community (Umeå Municipality, 2011, p. 7). In 2012, cooperation between social workers responsible for UASC, care home and supportive housing staff, legal guardians, and school representatives was organized into five networks (Hanberger et al., 2016). Issue-based cooperation was perceived as needed, as some questions and responsibilities "fell between the cracks." Cooperation concerning individual children did not work as well, for example, and some caregivers felt that different functions in the reception system and certain caregivers operated as "isolated islands." This reflects failure in providing good or integrated care, which, according to Tronto (2013), has five phases (i.e., caring about, caring for, caregiving, care-receiving, and caring with) that must be well coordinated (Tronto, cited in Zembylas, Bozalek, & Shefer, 2014). Cooperation within the accommodation chain worked fairly well early on, but not between the first and last links (the YMCA was an exception as it used the same staff throughout the reception and integration process).

Program Inclusiveness

The program (i.e., the reception system) can be developed *for*, *by*, and *with* the UASC—according to the DC perspective laid out before. Our evaluation revealed that the reception was mainly developed for the UASC, step by step from the bottom, by various caregivers and civil society groups. In addition, different caregivers involved the children in different ways and to different extents in the daily work and routines, indicating that the program was partly implemented with them.

Implications of the Chosen Evaluation and the Evaluator's Responsibilities

The evaluator's responsibilities, as discussed earlier, differ depending on which democracy perspective is adopted. A DC evaluator also has a responsibility to account for the local government's understanding of the problem and what is to be achieved. In this case, the local government adopted goals for the reception of UASC in 2006 (Umeå Municipality, 2006). In 2007, the city adopted a diversity policy to be implemented in all policy sectors, stating that Umeå should welcome everyone regardless of ethnicity, religion, or social background (Umeå Municipality, 2007). UASC should be ensured individual safety and safe accommodations, education, health and medical care, knowledge of culture and society, and active and meaningful social lives. In addition, they should be guaranteed an asylum process according to rule of law. The local government conceived the problem as a service delivery challenge: UASC should be provided the same conditions as all children living in Umeå. We see that the local government is taking a legal and organizational (versus a moral) responsibility approach to care, focusing on children's rights and security. This functional approach reflects a system-world perspective, that is, a rules-based framework with protocols, based on values such as accountability, productivity, efficiency, safety, and security, intended to protect and preserve the social order. Systems are helpful for issues that can be regulated by rules or involve the exchange of money. One may question whether systems are helpful in restoring the well-being and growth of the children, including their social integration. A democratic care perspective draws attention to the fact that the children could not meet ethnic Swedes as much as they wanted to, which impeded integration, and that decision-makers and many caregivers assumed a protective notion of good care.

Awareness in Democratic Caring Evaluation—Summing Up

A DC evaluator should develop competence to become aware of the matters discussed above, which are summarized in Box 4.1.

BOX 4.1 MATTERS TO BE AWARE OF IN DEMOCRATIC CARING EVALUATION

1. *Understandings of problems/challenges/needs*
   Describe understandings of problems/challenges/needs facing different care-receivers (expressed by the program and stakeholders)
2. *Conceptions of care-receivers*
   Describe conceptions of the care-receiver group and of individuals in need of care and support (expressed by the program and stakeholders)
3. *Care-receivers' values*
   Analyze care-receivers' values and how they perceive the new values to which they must adapt
4. *Notions of good care*
   Analyze notions of good care explicitly or implicitly expressed by caregivers, UASC, and other stakeholders
5. *Caregivers' roles and responsibility*
   Describe caregivers' formal/legal and functional adopted roles and responsibilities, as well as their moral responsibilities
6. *Caregivers' collective responsibilities*
   Describe caregivers' collective responsibilities and collaboration at different levels (e.g., the municipal, organizational, and grassroots levels)
7. *Caregivers' attitudes*
   Analyze caregivers' group and individual attitudes and understandings of care-receivers and their needs
8. *Program inclusiveness*
   Describe whether the program has been developed for, by, or with care-receivers
9. *Implications of chosen evaluation and the evaluator's responsibilities*
   Describe the aim and implications of the evaluation and the evaluator's responsibilities

Integration in a new society is another key issue in the case discussed. As the norms of the new society require attention, the evaluator needs knowledge of both cultural norms and multiculturalism (Hanberger, 2010). The latter is critical for reflecting on what sort of multicultural society a caring program promotes. A DC evaluation of the reception of UASC needs to be multiculturally aware, that is, consist of a culturally aware problem analysis including an understanding of power relations between minority groups and between these and the majority culture. Phillips (2007) is critical of policies that promote group rights, that is, that redistribute powers to cultural or religious groups. As Phillips emphasizes, men's power over women can be maintained by diversity policy and should therefore be attended to, but "regulation" as a policy option is insensitive to "differences in cultural norms and moral values" (2007, p. 160). Phillips' notion of multicultural awareness is in line with Tronto's notion of democratic care, and both should be considered matters to which a DC evaluator should be responsive in this case.

Some UASC have been socialized in cultures where honor is important and honored-related violence is accepted. Caregivers should be aware of this and what it means to grow up with different norms and loyalties, while taking action to socialize UASC into the majority culture's norms and fostering some kind of multicultural society. A DC evaluator needs to be multiculturally aware but not accepting of UASC who uphold norms that violate human rights and international laws (Hanberger, 2010).

The evaluator also needs to be responsive to changing conditions. In extraordinary situations, for example, when numerous UASC arrive, as in the fall of 2015 in many European countries, the challenges expand. In December 2015, Umeå had agreed to provide accommodations for at least 343 UASC per year compared with 40 in 2012. The evaluator should be responsive to the knowledge needs of stakeholders operating in rapidly changing environments and a highly polarized world.

Swedish reception of UASC is underpinned by international conventions on human rights, especially the Convention on the Rights of the Child (CRC). According to the CRC, the best interests of the child must be a primary consideration in all actions concerning children. When the reception system is under pressure, the evaluator should highlight when measures taken do not reflect the child's perspective and when children's needs are neglected. This implies supporting a generous and welcoming reception system, in which case the evaluator may be accused of bias by proponents of a more restrictive reception policy. Acting as a democratic evaluator in support of an elitist democracy can be criticized by advocates of discursive democracy and vice versa. Similarly, a DC evaluator conceiving good care as democratic care (Tronto's notion) can be questioned by evaluators conceiving good care as protective care. Furthermore, a multiculturally aware evaluator can be accused of bias by proponents of cultural coexistence if he or she regards cultural amalgamation as successful integration (Hanberger, 2010, p. 182).

CONCLUDING DISCUSSION

In democratic societies, citizens (e.g., voters, some care-receivers, and care-receivers' relatives), decision-makers (e.g., elected representatives in power and opposition), public administrators at various levels, and public and private caregivers have different functions and prescribed roles in policies and programs for people in need of care and support. Caring policies and programs often have generous and broad goals, but the preconditions for achieving them are not always provided, and care-receivers are generally in a weak position. This situation justifies developing DC evaluation to support a DC society welcoming various care-receivers. As demonstrated, there is more than one way to do this. The DC evaluator can start from different democratic evaluation orientations (i.e., elitist, participatory, or discursive) and different notions of good care, which will guide the evaluation in different directions. The UASC and their needs are perceived differently, for example, if caring is conceived from a protective or democratic care perspective (Tronto, 2016). As discussed above, DC evaluation does not refer to an entirely new evaluation approach and can be designed and implemented in several ways. The DC evaluation discussed here was developed within the discursive tradition, but not from House and Howe's (1999) framework. Integrating a caring commitment in the discursive democratic evaluation tradition entails more responsibility for vulnerable individuals and groups than does, for example, House and Howe's (1999) approach. If good and accountable care is conceived as situated in concrete situations for concrete people (Jerak-Zuiderent, 2015), the evaluation will pay more attention to local conditions, for example, how care quality and accountability are intertwined.

Acting as a DC evaluator in the case discussed here implies being aware of, and taking into account, the reception policy, the legal rights of UASC, the weak position of UASC as a group, and the individual children's specific needs. The evaluator also needs to be informed about various caregiver roles, views, and responsibilities and of the conditions under which caregivers operate, including power asymmetries. It is suggested that an evaluation intended to support a democratic and caring society should draw on knowledge from (discursive) democratic evaluation theory, research into good care, and research into the specific care-receivers in question. The matters a DC evaluator should be aware of have been summarized in Box 4.1. The contents of Box 4.1 can be used in two ways. First, the various matters can be kept in mind and applied in evaluating care policies and programs for different care-receivers. Second, the contents can also be applied in meta-evaluation of DC awareness in planned or finalized evaluations. Any DC evaluation will be informed by the cited research and pay more or less attention to the matters summarized in Box 4.1.

Issues to be aware of, and account for, in DC evaluation relate to what one conceives as the role of evaluation in a democratic society and the research used to inform the evaluation. The latter affects how care-receivers and their needs are conceived, and what is conceived as good care. The evaluator's role and responsibilities differ depending on the chosen evaluation approach and on whose knowledge needs it serves.

It is hoped that this chapter can inspire further discussion about what it means to develop evaluation in the service of a democratic and caring society, and what awareness, competencies, and responsibilities the evaluator needs to develop.

KEY CONCEPTS

- unaccompanied children
- elitist democratic evaluation
- participatory democratic evaluation
- discursive democratic evaluation
- stakeholders
- caregivers
- care-receivers
- good care
- evaluator's responsibilities

DISCUSSION QUESTIONS

1. It is recognized that program makers construct problems and design solutions in a policy discourse in which different perceptions of problems and solutions exist and compete. How the evaluator deals with this situation affects the legitimacy and credibility of the evaluation. *Whose perception of the problems should be addressed and accounted for in a DC evaluation? What perceptions of problems and care exist among program participants and come to dominate a program?*
2. Choosing a specific democratic evaluation approach entails ascribing different roles and responsibilities to the evaluator. Care-receivers are more or less able to participate in an evaluation, and we need to discuss to what extent different care-receivers can be involved in an evaluation. *Which democratic evaluation approach is*

most feasible to apply in evaluating programs for different care-receivers? How can care-receivers be included in the evaluation?

3. Evaluations that take account of theory of care (ethics) provide knowledge needed for understanding and managing problems and challenges encountered in caring programs. This chapter has offered some suggestions that theory on care (ethics) can apply, but the matter merits further discussion. *Which theories of good care are most relevant to evaluations of different care-receivers?*

REFERENCES

Abma, T., Leyerzapf, H., & Landeweer, E. (2016). Responsive evaluation in the interference zone between system and lifeworld. *American Journal of Evaluation, 38,* 507–520. doi:10.1177/1098214016667211

Carlson, B. E., Cacciatore, J., & Klimek, B. (2012). A risk and resilience perspective on unaccompanied refugee minors. *Social Work, 57,* 259–269.

Derluyn, I., & Broekaert, E. (2007). Different perspectives on emotional and behavioural problems in unaccompanied refugee children and adolescents. *Ethnicity and Health, 12,* 141–162.

Donabedian, A. (1988). The quality of care: How can it be assessed? *Archives of Pathology & Laboratory Medicine, 121,* 1145–1150.

Dryzek, J. S. (1996). *Democracy in capitalist times: Ideals, limits, and struggles.* New York, NY: Oxford University Press.

Dryzek, J. S. (2000). *Deliberative democracy and beyond: Liberals, critics, contestations.* Oxford, England: Oxford University Press.

Eriksson, M., Ghazinour, M., Hanberger, A., Isaksson, J., & Wimelius, M. (2013). *Utvärdering av insatser för ensamkommande flyktingungdomar i Umeå: Delrapport* [Evaluation of measures for unaccompanied minors in Umeå: Evaluation report]. Umeå, Sweden: Umeå University, Umeå Centre for Evaluation Research.

Eriksson, M., Ghazinour, M., Hanberger, A., Isaksson, J., & Wimelius, E. M. (2014). *Utvärdering av insatser för ensamkommande barn och ungdomar i Umeå 2012–2013: Slutrapport* [Evaluation of measures for unaccompanied minors in Umeå 2012–2013: Evaluation report]. Umeå, Sweden: Umeå University, Umeå Centre for Evaluation Research.

Farazmand, A. (1999a). Globalization and public administration. *Public Administration Review, 59,* 509–522.

Farazmand, A, (1999b). The elite question: Toward a normative elite theory of organization. *Administration & Society, 31,* 321–360.

Fazel, M., & Stein, A. (2002). The mental health of refugee children. *Archives of Disease in Childhood,* 87, 366–370.

Fekete, L. (2007). Detained: Foreign children in Europe. *Race & Class, 49,* 93–104.

Gutmann, A., & Thompson, D. (2004). *Why deliberative democracy?* Princeton, NJ: Princeton University Press.

Habermas, J. (1996). Three normative models of democracy. In S. Benhabib (Ed.), *Democracy and difference: Contesting the boundaries of the political* (pp. 21–30). Princeton, NJ: Princeton University Press.

Hanberger, A. (2001a). What is the policy problem? Methodological challenges in policy evaluation. *Evaluation, 7*, 45–62.

Hanberger, A. (2001b). Policy and program evaluation: Civil society and democracy. *American Journal of Evaluation, 22*, 211–228.

Hanberger, A. (2006). Evaluation of and for democracy. *Evaluation, 12*, 17–37.

Hanberger, A. (2010). Multicultural awareness in evaluation: Dilemmas and challenges. *Evaluation, 16*, 177–191.

Hanberger, A., Wimelius, M., Ghazinour, M., Isaksson, I., & Eriksson, M. (2016). Local service-delivery networks for unaccompanied children in Sweden: Evaluating their effectiveness. *Journal of Social Services Research, 42*, 675–688.

House, E. R., & Howe, K. R. (1999). *Values in evaluation and social research.* Thousand Oaks, CA: SAGE.

Ingvad, B. (2003). *Omsorg och relationer: Om det känslomässiga samspelet i hemtjänsten* [Care and relations: About the emotional interplay in home care]. (Doctoral dissertation). School of Social Work, Lund University, Lund, Sweden.

Jerak-Zuiderent, S. (2015). Accountability from somewhere and for someone: Relating with care. *Science as Culture, 24*, 412–435.

Kohli, R. K. S. (2011). Working to ensure safety, belonging and success for unaccompanied asylum-seeking children. *Child Abuse Review, 20*, 311–323.

MacDonald, B. (1976). Evaluation and the control of education. In D. A. Tawney (Ed.), *Curriculum Evaluation Today: Trends and Implications* (pp. 125–136). London, England: Macmillan.

Noddings, N. (1984). *Caring: A feminine approach to ethics and moral education.* Berkeley, CA: University of California Press.

Pateman, C. (1970). *Participation and democratic theory.* Cambridge, England: Cambridge University Press.

Phillips, A. (2007). *Multiculturalism without culture.* Princeton, NJ: Princeton University Press.

Picciotto, R. (2015). Democratic evaluation for the 21st century. *Evaluation, 21*, 150–166.

Shamseldin, L. (2012). Implementation of the United Nations Convention on the Rights of the Child 1989 in the care and protection of unaccompanied asylum seeking children: Findings from empirical research in England, Ireland and Sweden. *International Journal of Children's Rights, 20*(1), 90–121.

Schumpeter, J. (1942). *Capitalism, socialism and democracy.* New York, NY: Harper.

Szebehely, M., & Trydegård, G.-B. (2012). Home care for older people in Sweden: A universal model in transition. *Health & Social Care in the Community, 20*, 300–309.

Tronto, J. (1993). *Moral boundaries: A political argument for an ethic of care.* New York, NY: Routledge.

Tronto, J. C. (2014a). Moral boundaries after twenty years: From limits to possibilities. In G. Olthuis, H. Kohlen, & J. Heier (Eds.), *Moral boundaries redrawn: The significance of Joan Tronto's argument for political theory, professional ethics, and care as practice. Ethics of care,* Volume 3 (pp. 9–29). Leuven, Belgium: Peeters.

Tronto, J. C. (2014b). Ethics of care: Present and new directions. In G. Olthuis, H. Kohlen, & J. Heier (Eds.), *Moral boundaries redrawn: The significance of Joan Tronto's argument for political theory, professional ethics, and care as practice. Ethics of care,* Volume 3 (pp. 215–229). Leuven, Belgium: Peeters.

Tronto, J. (2016, September). *Protective care or democratic care? Some reflections on terrorism and care.* Presentation at SIGNAL, Cifas 23, Brussels, Belgium.

Umeå Municipality. (2006). *Verksamhetsplan—gruppboende för asylsökande barn och unga* [Work plan—housing facilities for asylum seeking minors]. Dnr. 280/2006. Umeå, Sweden: Umeå Municipality.

Umeå Municipality. (2007). *Protokoll 2007-06-18* [Minutes 2007-06-18]. [Minutes from Social and Welfare committee 2007-06-18] Umeå, Sweden: Author.

Umeå municipality. (2011). *Ensamkommande barn—ett gemensamt ansvar i Umeå* [Unaccompanied children—shared responsibility in Umeå]. Umeå, Sweden: Author.

United Nations High Commissioner for Refugees (UNHCR). (2012). *A year of crisis: Global Trends 2011.* Geneva, Switzerland: UNHCR.

United Nations High Commissioner for Refugees (UNHCR). (2014). *UNHCR Statistical Yearbook 2014* (14th ed.). Retrieved from http://www.unhcr.org/statistics/country/566584fc9/unhcr-statistical-yearbook-2014-14th-edition.html

Visse, M. A., Abma, T. A., & Widdershoven, G. A. M. (2015). Practising political care ethics: Can responsive evaluation foster democratic care? *Ethics and Social Welfare, 9,* 164–182.

Wærness, K. (1984). The rationality of caring. *Economic and Industrial Democracy, 5,* 185–211.

Widdershoven, G. A. M., & Huijer, M. (2001). The fragility of care: An encounter between Nussbaum's Aristotelian ethics and ethics of care. *International Journal in Philosophy and Theology,* 62, 304–316.

Zembylas, M., Bozalek, V., & Shefer, T. (2014). Tronto's notion of privileged irresponsibility and the reconceptualisation of care: Implications for critical pedagogies of emotion in higher education. *Gender and Education, 26,* 200–214.

PART III

ETHICS AND EVALUATION FOR A CARING SOCIETY

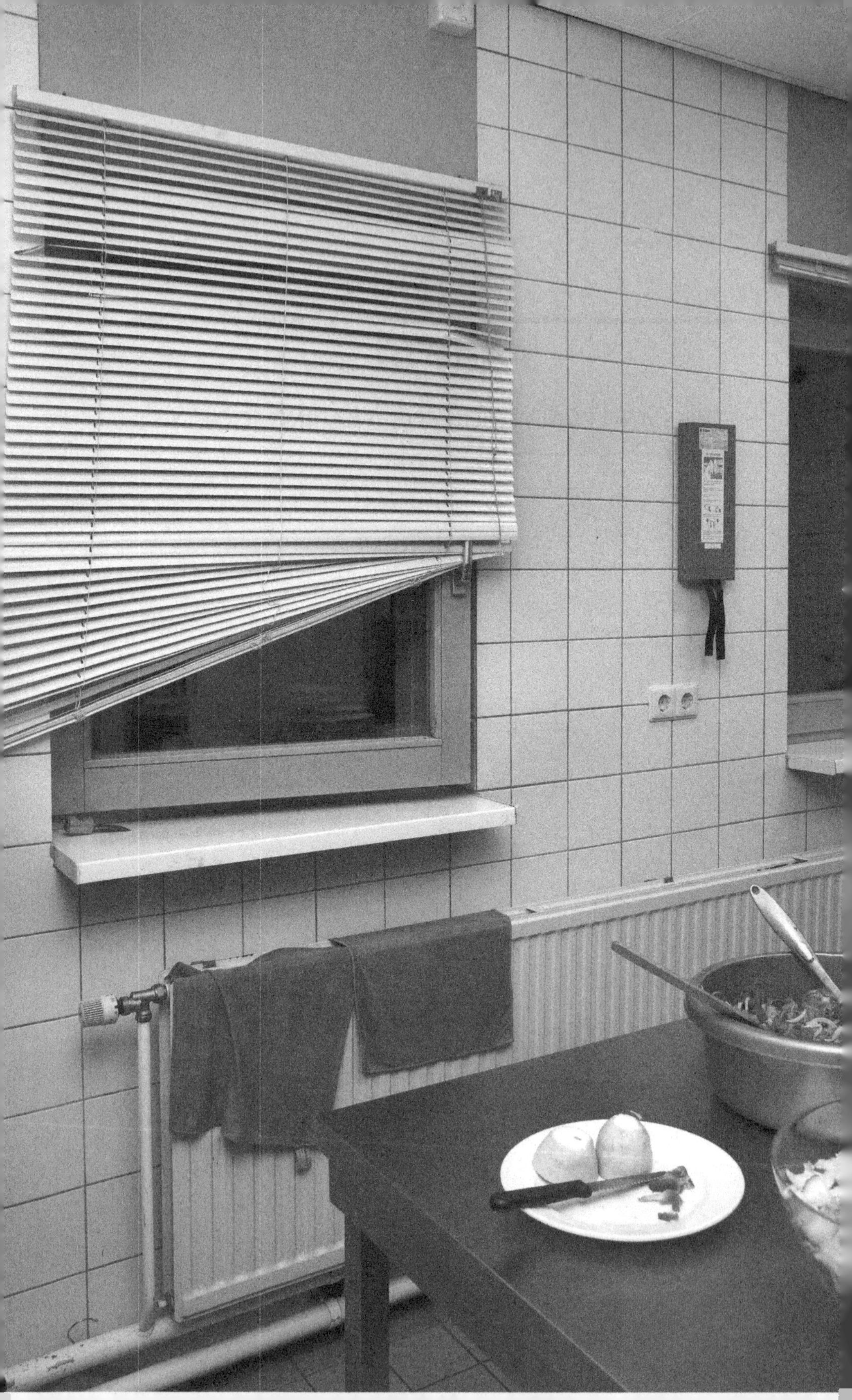

CHAPTER 5

UNCONTROLLED EVALUATION

The Case of Telecare Innovations

Jeannette Pols
University of Amsterdam

At the heart of evaluation is a set of criteria—too often implicit—that functions as a standard to which practices can be compared. These are usually criteria that can be operationalized and quantified. Examples are quality of life, self-management, and adherence to models or rules. Researchers often do not acknowledged the world of assumptions that underlie these evaluation studies and the criteria they use. Some of these assumptions are that interventions can be isolated from other events, and that these interventions have a causal, or at least highly probable, relationship to the effects observed. Researchers hardly ever question the idea that effects can be quantified and generalized over situations and populations (see Greenhalgh , Howick, & Maskrey, 2014; Mol & Karayalcin, 2008; Willems, Palmboom, & Lips, 2007 for critiques). Evaluation criteria incorporate moral ideas, for example, that criteria should be transparent so that those concerned know how something will be judged. As with school exams, those being tested should understand the criteria for testing.

Evaluation for a Caring Society, pages 127–140

Scholars engaged in qualitative evaluation have criticized fixed standards and predefined evaluation criteria. One of the well-known critiques is that knowing criteria in advance of an evaluation may lead to perverse effects. When organisations or individuals know they will be evaluated according to a particular criterion, they might work hard on this criterion, while neglecting others. An example is the constant complaints about delayed trains in the Netherlands, which led the government to formulate *punctuality targets.* The Dutch railway organisation implemented a new schedule to meet these, and punctuality increased. But this also meant that the passengers needed to cope with longer travel times, and more frequent changing of trains. This was not something the government or the travelers' organization had anticipated. Evaluation criteria hence shape what may be evaluated, which might be very different from improving a practice.

In this chapter I draw attention to a framework for evaluation that does not begin with preset criteria. This framework is designed to evaluate care programs, although it may have wider applicability. The framework constitutes a form of *evaluation in the wild,* meaning that it can be used outside the rigorously controlled laboratory conditions needed for quantitative evaluation. The idea is not only to counter perverse effects, although I will show some surprising examples of these as well. My aim is to draw attention to styles of evaluation that can take unexpected effects into account. I want to make space for open-ended questions—such as "What kind of effects emerge?"—that may bring forth new repertoires for understanding and improving care practices. Rather than objectifying practical achievements through the use of quantitative methods and outside standards, such an approach makes use of participants' practical knowledge and values they find meaningful. Evaluation in the wild adopts a collaborative approach (Marcus, 2013; Holmes & Marcus, 2008; Pols, 2004, 2008) that may lead to suggestions, sensitivities, and inspirations for improving care.

This book shows different approaches are possible to qualitative evaluation, rather than provide a single blueprint. In this chapter I build on work from the field of empirical ethics (see e.g., Pols, 2015; Willems & Pols, 2010; Willems, 2010; Mol, 2008, 2010; Thygesen & Moser, 2010). Empirical ethics research uses what I call the *loose concept*[1] of what Laurent Thévenot calls *forms of the good* (Thévenot, 2001). Empirical ethicists study what people aim to achieve and how they put different forms of the good into practice. The good is not only in the hearts and minds of people but is also embedded in technologies, rules, and institutions; as I will show, it also emerges in relationships among people and their social and material environment. What presents itself as good is then always something that needs to be specified and made concrete empirically.

Here I present an argument for evaluating care practices, although other normative practices may be studied from this point of view as well.[2] How does the analysis of different goods for different practices help to improve care practices (see also Mol, 2006; Moser, 2010)? This is, after all, the aim of evaluation: to look back and tease out the lessons that may be learned. I suggest that comparing practices, their embedded forms of goodness (and, for that matter, badness), and their effects form a powerful frame for this particular type of evaluation. By meticulously describing the conditions within which effects emerge, lessons can be transported to and applied in other places. What it means to "do good" is not static. It is a practical activity that combines good intentions with social and material specificities, and therefore demands ongoing evaluation.

Discerning ways of doing good in practice, then, does not mean that this good is beyond discussion. Normative orientations may work out differently, for different patient groups, for practices that are regulated differently, within differently oriented institutions, and so on. The evaluation work suggested here brings out the lessons that may be learned and specifies the conditions within which results may be transported elsewhere. This transportation demands active translations to learn if and how effects may be achievable elsewhere.

In this chapter I put some flesh on these theoretical bones by working through three examples of care practices that show how and where an empirical ethics perspective can be useful. I use insights gained from a series of studies of the use of telecare devices (Pols, 2012; Mort et al., 2015; López Gómez, 2015; Thygesen & Moser, 2010). There is a tremendous amount of technology evaluation studies being done using state-of-the-art quantitative measurements. What cannot be made visible using such methods, however, are the ways in which people *use* technology, and how they hence create new values and knowledge. What problems do they solve with the technology, and what values do they enact in doing so? The examples I use I take from my book *Care at a Distance* (Pols, 2012). They serve to illustrate the possibilities for qualitative evaluation in the wild, or what I dubbed in the book *uncontrolled field studies* (see Pols, 2012, Chapter 8).

THE SATURATION METER

My first example is the use of a blood saturation meter. What happens when a simple device is put into practice? Blood saturation meters measure the amount of oxygen in the blood. If there is too little oxygen in the blood, tissues may not get enough and may be damaged. Obviously, this is to be avoided. I studied the use of the saturation meter in a rehabilitation clinic for people with severe chronic obstructive pulmonary disease (COPD, to some better known by its old name of lung emphysema). This is a disease that is typical for mine workers and heavy smokers. The elasticity of the lungs is damaged, and this causes difficulty taking up oxygen, which causes people with COPD to get out of breath quickly when they exert themselves. The people in the clinic were often very ill, and could not walk much—sometimes not even 50 meters—before getting short of breath. Their everyday life was seriously jeopardized by the disease. They were in the clinic to learn how to live with the disease, supported by a multidisciplinary team that approached this task from different angles.

So what could a blood saturation meter do in this practice? Take a minute to imagine possible effects. Could it support self-management? Improve quality of life? Or could it be a kind of personal alarm system? These imaginings already show that a device needs to be understood—and used!—in relation to particular aims and activities. These practices are important for the question of how to evaluate the use of a device like a saturation meter. Let's see how this worked out in the rehabilitation clinic and at home, as one patient, Mrs. Jarmus explained why the saturation meter was difficult to use:

Mrs. Jarmus: You see, I had to learn to walk slowly, right from the start, walk very slowly. It doesn't come naturally to me. And then I used the saturation device and I noticed that after walking a minute, my saturation level goes down, or it drops below 90, and then I have to stop. So, well . . . a minute is not long.

Jeannette: So you walk a minute and then take a one-minute break?

Mrs. Jarmus: Yes, that's it. But I find it so hard to put into practice! You have to stop in front of every shop window, look as if you're very interested in something, when there's nothing to see! Play with your car keys or whatever. And sometimes you just can't do even that. I have days when I can hardly get from the kitchen to the sofa.

Mrs. Jarmus had to put the saturation meter and the knowledge it brings to good use. She had to translate it to link it to a practice. She made a first translation from oxygen saturation to time: After one minute of very slow walking, she should stop. The indication of 90% saturation then is a directive: "rest one minute." Then she made another translation; one minute's rest meant a concrete practice one minute of standing still. This was easily done on the grounds of the clinic, but back home it was more awkward to do so in public, in an everyday situation where people hardly ever stand still. It was on the streets where people watch you, and that made standing still quite a different and much more difficult job.

The body changed with each translation Mrs. Jarmus made. Each body had its own troubles and possible solutions. The first body was a body with blood that contains oxygen that may sink to a level that is too low to keep moving without damage to tissues. This body became a body that should rest after one minute of walking. The body needing rest became a body that is visible to others. It stood inexplicably inert in public places. This body needed to learn how to rest inconspicuously in public space.

The example shows that any technology is not something in and of itself, but obtains meaning through particular practices. Rather than simply deliver what is expected, technology use needs translation and practical contextualisation. This brings new problems with it and demands new skills to solve these. If one wants to evaluate the use of the saturation meter in the care of people with COPD, these translations are important to take into account. It can, however, rarely be predicted in advance how people will make these translations. These need to be established by observing how technologies work in practice and how their users make them useful. One could say that the saturation meter does not simply "have an effect," as a discrete intervention, like 100 mg of a certain drug, would. Its meaningful use would demand, for example, training in walking and standing still in the streets. An exchange of practical knowledge and skills developed for doing this might be valuable. In this embedded way, saturation meters can be seen to gain an effect, or more precisely, help establish new relations between people, their diseases, and their daily lives. Rather than evaluating the saturation meter from a distance, close observation and discussion fits better as a way to learn from this care practice and transport its lessons to elsewhere.

There are of course different ways to tackle a saturation level that is too low. Giving Mrs. Jarmus a mobility scooter would have led to a very different series of translations in her situation. What needs to be evaluated then is the desirability of these different ways of living with disease *and* with devices. Should one practice walking and resting, or give up on walking altogether? These are not simply medical decisions. They invoke considerations about what constitutes a good life.

THE SAME TECHNOLOGY?

My second example shows how the same device may have different identities for different users and other people concerned. The case, involving the *telekit* comprised of a laptop with webcam and chat facility, is again from the rehabilitation clinic for patients with COPD and asthma, and is analyzed in detail in Pols and Willems (2011). The example shows that establishing routines for the use of a technology may become confused because the same technology has different identities for different users. What the technology is and how it is supposed to support particular aims of care differ for different people, as do activities to use it efficiently. In this case, such differences in identity caused miscommunications that the participants could not untangle; these became apparent in discussions about how long the patients should use the telekit.

In this study, participants used the telekit for 3 months to speak by video call with their caregivers in the clinic and to communicate with former fellow patients. At the time of the study, managers, technicians, and caregivers were discussing the future of the telekit. In their deliberations over how to evaluate the telekit and its potential uses, opposing ideas on what care is and what it should be about were articulated. The telekit had two identities, each related to different treatment goals and routines for efficient use. The first identity related to the goal of guaranteeing the effect of the treatment. This turned out to demand very different routines compared to the second notion of what the telekit should do—providing a "window on the world." Based on these different treatment goals, the clinical staff and the managers described the identity of the telekit using two metaphors: as a digital umbilical cord connecting the patient to the clinic or as an inhaler providing the needed "puff" to get on with life.

The Telekit as an Umbilical Cord

When the caregivers formulated the purpose of the telekit as "to consolidate the effect of the treatment," proponents intended it to help patients develop adequate behavior to cope with their illness. This meant that patients had to put into practice what they had learned in the clinic. The telekit directly relates to, and stands in the service of, the work done in the clinic. Here the metaphor for the telekit is the umbilical cord that attaches the patient to the clinic and allows them to be "fed" more of the clinic's wisdom. In this view, contact with the principal caregivers, social workers, was central to telekit use. The principal caregiver was supposed to check on patients, discuss their problems with them, and encourage them to take the steps laid down in the treatment plan that they had made together in the clinic. Contact with the social worker guaranteed the continuity of the work done in the clinic.

Contact with former fellow patients would serve the same purpose: to bridge the gap between clinic and home by exchanging advice on how to cope. Three months of computer use should then be sufficient to reach these goals. Patients were supposed to become independent of the clinic and its devices—using the telekit enough to become independent of it—with the telekit remaining in the realm of the clinic. If patients wanted to go on using computers after the umbilical cord was severed, this was encouraged (and indeed trained for) in the clinic. However, the clinic would not be providing the hardware. People would have to buy their own computers, just as they would have to join their local sports clubs and rely on care from their own specialists and home caregivers. Hence, use of email and the internet was seen as ambiguously both part and not part of the treatment.

In the end, the proper way to deal with umbilical cords is to cut them, when the attached one has other, more grown up resources and means to feed themselves independently. This is a specific notion of treatment as "a temporary intervention by professionals," in which the professionals are supposed to make themselves superfluous. Treatment has to stop, and people have to learn how to fend for themselves with the help of their local caregivers. They have to cut themselves free of the clinic.

The Telekit as an Inhaler

If the telekit was intended, instead, to provide patients with a window on the world, the telekit mainly became a device to actively continue the tasks set in the clinic and get on with life better. One problem patients have, for instance, is social isolation and a dearth of meaningful activities; they do not have much to do with their day, as their mobility is gravely impaired. Many had had trouble leaving the house, and they learned solutions for this in the clinic, such as establishing an active social network with fellow patients. Fellow patients could become friends or close acquaintances connected by webcam, and provide enduring support and company.

Internet and email use were important in this telekit framing. Patients need to employ both as structural ways of seeking entertainment and keeping in touch. The internet connection supported such services as online shopping, gaming, entertainment, and social media. The telekit thus became a structural part of the social, practical, and emotional life of patients, facilitating many different contacts after leaving the clinic. The device supported patients in building their new world.

One of my informants compared the telekit to an inhaler, a device that COPD patients use continually to counter breathlessness. But if the telekit is like an inhaler, patients are dependent on it, making it rather cruel to withdraw the device after 3 months. It would be like giving a person a wheelchair—or indeed an inhaler—and then taking it away even if the need for it has not disappeared. People do not have to emancipate from the device, but should use the telekit structurally, as useful and dependable technology. In this case, the telekit is a permanent aid rather than a temporary lifeline.

Whether the telekit was an umbilical cord or an inhaler, the clinic's care would not be permanent. Patients had to cut themselves free of the professionals, even though some thought this was indeed a pity. But they did not have to part with online communication, which was ongoing as patients used the new device to reshape their world, making it part of the everyday muddle of getting through the day and facing new problems. The telekit functioned as an inhaler rather than as an umbilical cord.

Routines and Identities

The two identities of the telekit meant two sets of routines, implying two ways of organising care at home efficiently. The double identity of the device and its use were not explicit. Both scenarios were present at the same time, with the caregivers unaware of the differences. That they held different views on treatment was something they had not come up against before. The technology simultaneously materialized and separated the different goals that the caregivers were already accommodating. On the one hand, treatment should have the effect of helping people find meaningful connections to the world. On the other hand, practicing what one has learned during treatment is a way of engaging with the world. The telekit differentiated these aims by separating the different sets of routines patients needed to employ to achieve either goal.

In the daily telekit operations, the different sets of routines were tacitly present, with sometimes one or the other in the foreground. On a theoretical level, the two ways of caring and using the telekit were different, but in practice they were mixed up, muddling discussions and complicating practices. The case shows that evaluating a technology is complex because there may be different understandings of what a technology is, why people should use it, and how to use it efficiently. Both goods imagined for the telekit seem valid. Both treatment effects—consolidation of treatment effects as well as adding meaning to life—are important and overlapping assignments for patients. Any state-of-the-art evaluation must embed its own understanding of a device and its anticipated effects. The first evaluative step could be to uncover these practical understandings, figure out how to think about these different uses, and determine which one should be supported.

DISTURBING EVALUATIONS

My last example addresses the well recognized—if rarely remedied—effect that the practice of evaluating itself interferes with the very practice being studied. Innovative care practices can be seen as sites of construction. Ideally, research should not hinder this construction work in order to not disturb or harm the innovations. This is difficult for state-of-the-art quantitative research, which needs to construct their own workplace in order to create the conditions for good research. Conditions need to be standardized, patients need to be randomly assigned to experimental and control groups, questionnaires need to be filled out by caregivers and patients, and so on. Often, nurses caring for patients also collect data for research. Apart from caring for their patients or tinkering with devices, I found that nurses come to care for telecare systems' administration and their evaluation. They adjusted patient files, sent faxes, consulted technicians in order to make devices work.

In one example, caregivers had to offer a telecare device to all patients in the clinic, even if they knew the device would be of no use to some of them. They had to do this to follow research methods—based on randomized controlled clinical trials—designed to objectively establish who would benefit from telecare and who would not. This standard for good research was in tension with understandings of good care. Good research and good care have different requirements. This often leads to compromises in care research, making quantitative research less viable in care practices. Because it may disturb care practices unduly, randomisation is often not attempted. Small numbers of patients, difficulties in recruiting them, and ethical reasons also stand in the way of randomisation. When data collectors and caregivers are the same people, they need to make constant trade-offs between rigorously standardized research and individual patient care.

The interdependence of research practices and the projects they evaluate is particularly problematic in research into innovative technology. When a telecare project depends on research infrastructure, the care practice stops at the same time the research stops. No data are collected anymore. Waiting for the results begins. When results arrive, they are often ambiguous and need to be processed by the proper bureaucracies. If the project lacks finances for continuation and the results are ambivalent, the telecare practice fades out before any decision is taken. This *project nature* (see Law, 1994 for this term) of telecare innovation seems to be a public secret around telecare, as Langstrup-Nielsen (2005), and Finch, May, Mair, Mort, and Gask (2003) also describe. It is both *public* because all concerned know it happens like this and *secret* because it continues to be common practice. Innovative projects come and go, and research chapters pile up, without long-term effects on care practice.

However sad this situation may be, for this chapter it is important to see how evaluation is a practice in itself, one that may interfere with the very innovations it wants to evaluate. The perverse effects, if one wants to use that term, do not emerge from the criteria formulated, but from the practices needed to structure particular forms of research. Two construction sites interfere, that of the innovative care practice and that of the research. Both construction sites aim to build different edifices; they sometimes support each other, and at other times a choice has to be made for building one or the other. In the research construction site, interventions should not be tinkered with, or the intervention Mrs. Jarmus got would be different from the one given Mrs. Pietersen. The research would then evaluate different interventions and become useless. For the care practices construction site, adapting interventions would improve care, for instance allowing caregivers to judge whom of their patients might benefit from it. Construction sites of care and quantitative research intersect and collide because they have different objectives.[3] It is difficult to combine state-of-the-art quantitative research with state-of-the-art care while using the same infrastructures.[4]

The qualitative evaluation studies presented in this volume do not intrude on care practices, not by pre-defining the object of study nor by disturbing it. Certainly, an evaluator hanging around and wanting to engage in conversations takes up caregivers' time. But because it can be done in the field, this type of evaluation can go with the flow rather than divert care's rhythms. Evaluation in the wild can make use of locally developed knowledge about work practices and take unexpected findings into account.

CONCLUSIONS

Technology's effects on care practices may be unpredictable due to translations that need to be made to put a technology to practical use. This is one of the reasons why so much research being done on technology teaches us so little. Translation processes are not taken into account because criteria to judge success are predefined in quantitative types of evaluation. The examples presented here show how different understandings and uses of a technology might pose a problem for evaluation, as one or the other may be inscribed in the evaluation's definition of outcome variables. Controlled studies of care practices need to build, so to speak, a laboratory in the field, and this may disturb care practices in the evaluation process.

Qualitative evaluation studies provide interesting alternatives to avoid these problems. Their focus is on how exactly the object of research takes shape (good care, use of technology, and values strived for). Rather than measuring the occurrence of something that is framed by the research protocol, these studies take ways of framing and enacting as the object of study itself. In this way actual use practices come into focus and lessons may be learned from pioneers, based on the knowledge gained through their practices and the values they achieved. The pragmatics of technology use can be made visible and useful to others. Rather than asking: "Does this technology work?" The question becomes: "*How* does this technology work within the relations it is put to use?" In this way the unexpected can find its place in our evaluation studies. Research may venture into the wild, to study practices as they unfold, without imposing definitions or infrastructures. We may expect the unexpected rather than trying to define and tame it.[5]

To what type of lessons can this type of research lead? There are some generalities to be learned from comparative studies on technology in care. The first is that many telecare devices are being developed and implemented that focus on the transportation of information, the "I" in ICT. Without exception, however, patients and informal caregivers value devices that support the "C" of communication (see Thygesen & Pols, 2106; Pols, 2012, Chapters 4 & 5 for examples). Taking this finding seriously would have a far-reaching impact on policies and industries that promote technology for solving the problems of an ageing society. Cost reduction through increased self-management of patients is the promised outcome. However, the notion of self-management frames people in individualized models of self care. In our research, patients and informal caregivers were more interested in creating supportive (digital) networks to get advice and support. Rather than managing alone, people look for support and advice. This demands different types of technology as well as different aims for health care policy. Different devices do different things, while people do different things with devices. Such "use practices" can be made visible in uncontrolled field studies.

To understand the workings of technology, we may need to uncover the new relationships it helps establish between the actors concerned, ranging from organisations working together, to patients, families, and nurses collaborating to implement a device (Pols, 2015). Each partner tries to nudge the others into a use practice that is desirable to their particular needs. The multitude of actors and the lack of knowledge about local concerns make telecare innovations unpredictable at best, and unsuccessful at worst. It is crucial to take these processes into account when one wants to evaluate a technology.

This means that the complexity and fragility of "doing good" in practice becomes visible, both for caregivers and for researchers. Often in care, there are no quick fixes and values may contradict one another. Annemarie Mol (2010) shows, for instance, how different efforts to achieve some form of the good may contradict one another; these tensions are not solved, but coexist, demanding persistent improvisation and tinkering from caregivers. Attempts at doing good are often processes of negotiation, adjusting and adapting in response to new situations, opportunities, and complications. Rather than delivering purportedly stable evidence, qualitative evaluation studies in the wild may make these tensions and processes visible. Recognising these may lead to suggestions, tools, and sensitivities that themselves need continuing reflection and adaptation to make them useful within local circumstances.

KEY CONCEPTS

- Empirical ethics
- Care ethics
- Evaluation
- Innovation
- Technology
- "Loose concept of the good"
- The unexpected
- Comparison

DISCUSSION QUESTIONS

1. How do you perceive the interference and collision of innovative care practices and evaluation?
2. The author stresses the importance of studying practices as they *unfold* and advises readers to expect the unexpected. What would that mean for evaluation methodologies? How would we assess the quality of the evaluation?
3. Empirical ethicists study what people aim to achieve and how they put different forms of the good into practice. How do you think their aim and activities differ from those of other researchers?

NOTES

1. Loose concepts steer one's gaze, but need empirical concretisation.
2. There is a recent attention to the normativity in scientific practices (e.g., Puig delaBellacasa, 2011).
3. For an analysis of how the clinical trial is an intervention in a particular form of life, see Dehue, 2001, 2002. Rather than *mirroring nature* to present the facts, it is an intervention in a practice. For a critique on the metaphor of mirroring, see Rorty, 1979. An innovative technology such as telecare cannot be regarded as a finite intervention that has predetermined types of effects that may be assessed in standard research (see also: May & Ellis, 2001; Lehoux et al., 2002).
4. See Langstrup, 2013 for the notion of care infrastructures.
5. Janelle Taylor puts the problems and possibilities of doing this nicely into context in her 2014 chapter.

REFERENCES

de la Bellacasa, M. P. (2011). Matters of care in technoscience: Assembling neglected things. *Social Studies of Science, 41*(1), 85–106.

Dehue, T. (2001). Establishing the experimenting society: The historical origin of social experimentation according to the randomized controlled design. *American Journal of Psychology, 114*(2), 283.

Dehue, T. (2002). A Dutch treat: Randomized controlled experimentation and the case of heroin-maintenance in the Netherlands. *History of the Human Sciences, 15*(2), 75–98.

Finch, T., May, C., Mair, F., Mort, M., & Gask, L. (2003) Integrating service development with evaluation in telehealthcare: an ethnographic study. *British Medical Journal, 327,* 1205–1209.

Greenhalgh, T., Howick, J., & Maskrey, N. (2014). Evidence based medicine: A movement in crisis? *BMJ, 348,* g3725.

Holmes, D. R., & Marcus, G. E. (2008). Collaboration today and the re-imagination of the classic scene of fieldwork encounter. *Collaborative Anthropologies, 1*(1), 81–101.

Langstrup, H. (2013). Chronic care infrastructures and the home. *Sociology of Health and Illness, 35*(7), 1008–1022.

Langstrup-Nielsen, H. L. (2005). *Linking healthcare—An inquiry into the changing performances of web-based technology for asthma monitoring.* PhD thesis, Copenhagen Business School.

Law, J. (1994). *Organizing modernity.* Oxford, England: Blackwell.

Lehoux, P., Sicotte, C., Denis, J.-L., Berg, M., & Lacroix, A. (2002). The theory of use behind telemedicine: How compatible with physicians' clinical routines? *Social Science and Medicine, 54*(6), 889–904.

López Gómez, D. (2015). Little arrangements that matter: Rethinking autonomy-enabling innovations for later life. *Technological Forecasting and Social Change, 93,* 91–101. doi:10.1016/j.techfore.2014.02.015

Marcus, G. (2013). Experimental forms for the expression of norms in the ethnography of the contemporary. *HAU: Journal of Ethnographic Theory, 3*(2), 197–217.

May, C., & Ellis, N. T. (2001). When protocols fail: Technical evaluation, biomedical knowledge, and the social production of 'facts' about a telemedicine clinic. *Social Science and Medicine, 53*(8), 989–1002.

Mol, A. (2006). Proving or improving: On health care research as a form of self-reflection. *Qualitative Health Research, 16*(3), 405–414.

Mol, A. (2008). *The logic of care: Health and the problem of patient choice.* London, England: Routledge.

Mol, A. (2010). Care and its values: Good food in the nursing home. In A. Mol, I. Moser, & J. Pols (Eds.), *Care in practice: On tinkering in clinics, homes and farms* (pp. 215–234). Bielefeld, Germany: Transcript Verlag.

Mol, A., & Karayalcin, C. (2008). "Evidence" is niet genoeg: Kanttekeningen uit de praktijk van de acute psychiatrie ["Evidence" is not enough. observations from the practice of acute psychiatry]. *Tijdschrift voor Psychiatrie, 50*(6), 359–364.

Mort, M., Roberts, C., Pols, J., Domenech, M., & Moser, I. (2015). Ethical implications of home telecare for older people: A framework derived from a multisited participative study. *Health Expectations, 18*(3), 438–449. doi:10.1111/hex.12109

Moser, I. (2010). Perhaps tears should not be counted but wiped away: On quality and improvement in dementia care. In A. Mol, I. Moser, & J. Pols (Eds.), *Care in practice: On tinkering in clinics, homes and farms* (pp. 277–300). Bielefeld, Germany: Transcript Verlag.

Pols, J. (2004). *Good care: Enacting a complex ideal in long-term psychiatry.* Utrecht, Netherlands: Trimbos-insituut.

Pols, J. (2008). Which empirical research, whose ethics? Articulating ideals in long-term mental health care. In G. Widdershoven, J. MacMillan, T. Hope, & L. Scheer (Eds.), *Empirical Ethics in Psychiatry* (pp. 51–68). Oxford, England: Oxford University Press.

Pols, J. (2012). How to make your relationships work? Aesthetic relations with technology. *Foundations of Science, 22*(2), 421–424.

Pols, J. (2015). Towards an empirical ethics in care: Relations with technologies in health care. *Medicine, Health Care, and Philosophy, 18*(1), 81–90. doi:10.1007/s11019-014-9582-9

Pols, J., & Willems, D. (2011) Innovation and evaluation. Taming and unleashing telecare technologies. *Sociology of Health & Illness, 33*(4), 484–498.

Rorty, R. (1979). *Philosophy and the mirror of nature.* Princeton, NJ: Princeton University Press.

Taylor, J. S. (2014). The demise of the bumbler and the crock: From experience to accountability in medical education and ethnography. *American Anthropologist, 116*(3), 523–534.

Thévenot, L. (2001). Pragmatic regimes governing the engagement with the world. In T. Schatzki, K. Knorr-Cetina, & E. von Savigny (Eds.), *The practice turn in contemporary theory* (pp. 56–73). London, England: Routledge.

Thygesen, H., & Moser, I. (2010). Technology and good dementia care: an argument for an ethics-in-practice approach. In M. Schillmeier & M. Domènech (Eds.), *New technologies and emerging spaces of care* (pp. 129–147). Farnham, England: Ashgate.

Thygesen, H., & Pols, J. (2016). 8.1 Care, Self-Management and the Webcam. In L. Manderson, E. Cartwright, & A. Hardon (Eds.), *The Routledge Handbook of Medical Anthropology* (p. 166). London, England: Routledge.

Willems, D. (2010). Varieties of goodness in high-tech home care. In A. Mol, I. Moser, & J. Pols (Eds.), *Care in practice: On tinkering in clinics, homes and farms* (pp. 257–276). Bielefeld, Germany; Transcript Verlag.

Willems, D., & Pols, J. (2010). Goodness! The empirical turn in health care ethics. *Issues,* 1, 1.

Willems, D., Vos, R., Palmboom, G., & Lips, P. (2007). *Passend bewijs: Ethische vragen bij het gebruik van evidence in het zorgbeleid* [Evidence that fits: Ethical questions for the use of evidence in care policy]. Den Haag, Netherlands: Centrum voor Ethiek en Gezondheid.

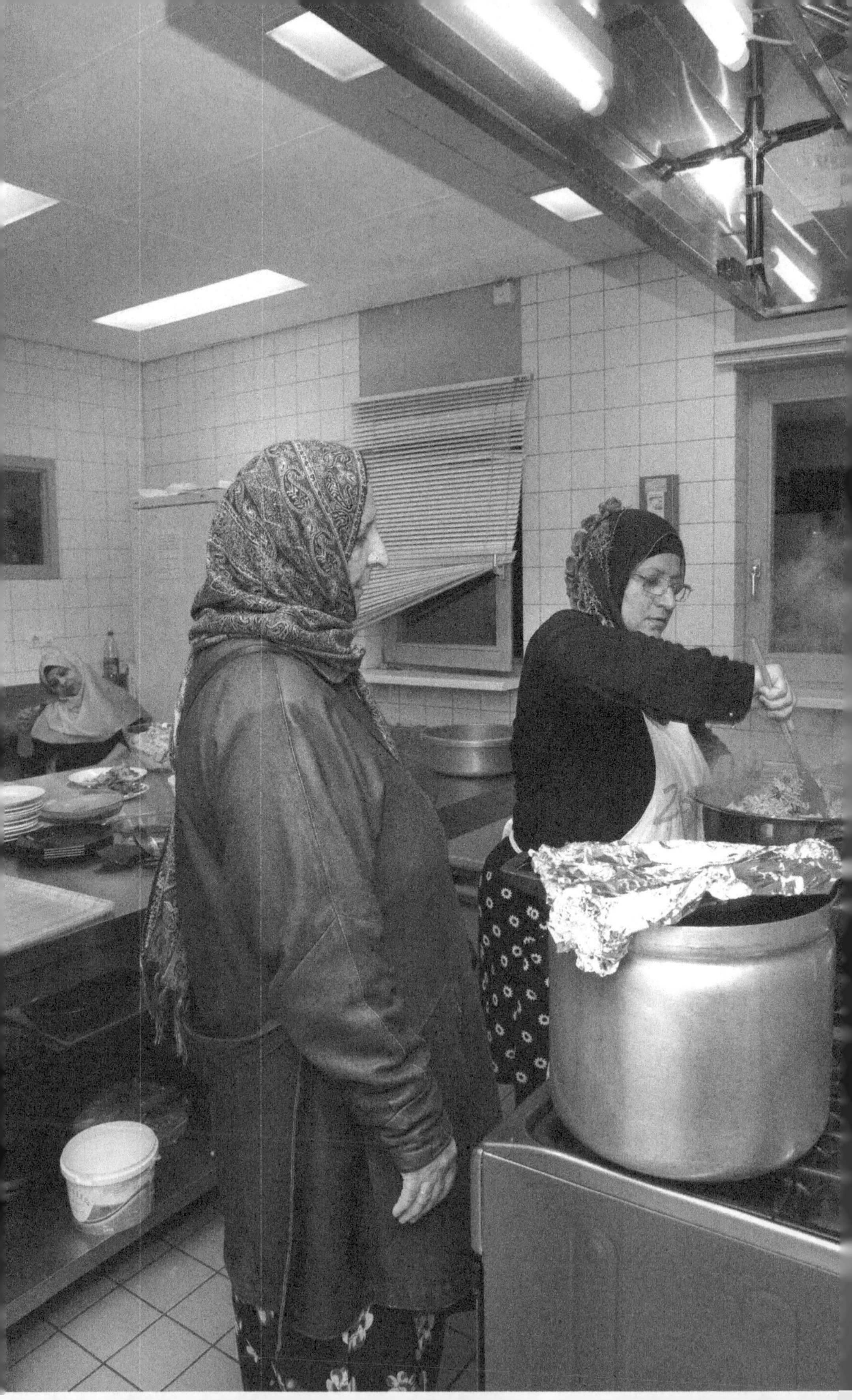

CHAPTER 6

EVALUATION FOR MOVING ETHICS IN HEALTH CARE SERVICES TOWARDS DEMOCRATIC CARE

A Three Pillars Model: Education, Companionship, and Open Space

Helen Kohlen
University of Vallendar

In Germany within the last 20 years, like in other European countries, an increasing number of ethical consultation services has been organized in hospitals, recently also in nursing homes. Organizational forms of ethics in health care institutions like hospital ethics committees (HEC) have become a criterion to fulfil quality standards in accreditation processes. Health care services try to meet the quality standards and see what it implies for an implementation. Moreover, some health care services try to work on an individual model that shows how the standard is put into practice in their particular institution. The Paul Gerhardt Diaconia (PGD), a nonprofit health

Evaluation for a Caring Society, pages 143–155

care service, has taken the step of developing a model of doing and moving ethics in the sense of actively trying to move forward any kind of attempt of organizing clinical ethics by analysing what has turned out to be fruitful and what has not turned out to be fruitful for everyday practices. Since the research is focusing the work of practitioners, their involvement in the organisation of ethics and finding ways how to empower them, an action research design was chosen.

Action research as a form of emancipatory research with a long tradition in community as well as organizational development work can meet the purpose of the study: exploring ways of organizing ethics and empowering practitioners (Hart & Bond, 1998). The overall question of the action research project is: "How should clinical ethics be organized to meet the needs of clinical professional actors, patients, and their families?" In this article professional actors are put into focus. In the process of creating a model that meets the needs, evaluations by all actors included took place during the whole project.

This undertaking is theoretically informed by political care ethics. It puts a relational perspective at the forefront and aims towards practices of democratic care. Especially in (German) health care institutions, care work is still ordered in a very hierarchical way and any movement towards democratic care can only be realized along extended pathways. Putting political care ethics into action means working with plurality of values and interests, engaging asymmetrical power relationships, and facing conflicts. Anchored in a relational and hermeneutic perspective, methodologically, an action research approach with a maximum of participation of actors in the field was developed.

Based on a maximum of involvement and participation of the Paul Gerhardt Diaconia (PGD) professional health care actors (practitioners) between 2010 and 2012, the democratic model of doing and moving ethics has been created. The participatory approach aims to bring in diverse voices and multiple perspectives. The circling processes of learning and changing practices address the move of ethics in three dimensions: education, companionship, and open space. In the language of practitioners the model consists of three pillars: (a) ethics education, (b) companionship and team development, and (c) open space meetings. Interactivity and a lively network of learning communities has been key in the whole process to link the pillars to each other. For making the process work as a movement towards democratic care, the building of trust and fostering a continuity of communication characterized by respect for plurality were decisive. In this chapter, I will present the model and how it has been developed within a participatory action research project as an ongoing process of (self-) evaluation.

THE PGD HEALTH CARE ENTERPRISE, DOING ETHICS AND PROBLEM IDENTIFICATION

The PGD is a nonprofit health care service named after the Lutheran theologian Paul Gerhardt (1607–1676) who became famous for his writing of hymns. The PGD health care service consists of eight hospitals, seven nursing homes, seven ambulatory home care services, two palliative care home services, and one hospice. Most of their care service is situated in Berlin. The total number of patients is about 85,000, the number of beds 1,400, and of employees 4,800. An Academy in Lutherstadt Wittenberg was opened in 2009 to offer further education for all employees who express their educational needs that help to identify an employee-oriented program each year anew. Classes in ethics education are included.

The initiative to put clinical ethics in motion was taken by the board of directors in 2009. Hospital Ethics Committees were implemented in some of the hospitals, but there was no transparency about what they were actually doing, what kind of challenges they were facing, and what kind of support would help them in their development and empowerment. The board had an interest in gaining an overview of the activities on ethics, current developments, and seeing opportunities of connectedness between the committees. Moreover, the following questions were raised: "What has to be done with regard to the hospitals, nursing homes, home care services, and hospices that are in the beginning stage of building up an organizational form of doing ethics?" and "What has to be done with regard to those parts of the organization that have not even started on this initiative?"

BRINGING IN POLITICAL CARE ETHICAL PERSPECTIVES

In 2010 a participatory action research project was designed with the intention of developing a program that would empower professional health care actors to move ethics in practice by bringing in care ethical perspectives. An attention to care ethics in the hospital arena was brought about by the findings of a research project that investigated into the history and practices of hospital ethics committees: The constant use of a principle-based approach revealed a technical language that dismissed or marginalized issues of care, especially with regard to questions end-of-life care. A lack of personnel, competencies, rooms, and unclear responsibilities were identified as reasons that caused ethical problems in the first place and missed care out (Kohlen, 2009a).

Merel Visse and her colleagues (2015) clearly describe: "Care is more than a virtue, bound to persons. Ontologically care ethics as a political ethics is grounded in a relational paradigm that honors interdependence in caring relationships and the constant changes in positions of vulnerability and fragility" (p. 167). Using a language of care by drawing on political care ethical theories, not only the importance of relatedness, the necessity of attentiveness to needs, competence and responsiveness can be made visible, but also conflicts, matters of power relationships and questions of responsibilities (Conradi, 2001; Tronto, 1993; Urban Walker, 1998).

PUTTING THE IDEA OF A CARING DEMOCRACY INTO THE HEALTH CARE ARENA

From a sociopolitical perspective, care is seen as a "collective and political practice that builds up society" (Nistelrooij, 2014, p. 39). Selma Sevenhuijsen (1996) has developed the idea of a transformative approach to share care work in society by seeing its value for and by everyone. She (1998) argues that care requires commitments to plurality, communication, trust, and respect. Tronto (2013) highlights that these qualities help to explain what the critical moral qualities are that will make it possible for people to take collective responsibility and to think of being both, a receiver and giver of care. In Tronto's (2013) vision, a caring democracy should also meet three requirements: (a) freedom that implies an absence of domination, (b) equality in order to support equal voice, and (c) justice to allow a process of assigning responsibilities and doing inclusion. The commitments to plurality, communication, trust, and respect help acting in solidarity, what Tronto calls "caring with" (2013, p. 35).

Within daily caring practices, like in health care institutions, relationships between people vary according to less and more powerful roles and positions, as well as changes in states of being more or less vulnerable, resilient, and fragile (Kohlen, 2014). The complexity of care and the dynamic caused by constant changes require reflective spaces within which to make decisions that might only count for a couple of days, sometimes only hours, until the revisiting of current states and events are necessary.

Avishai Margalit (1997) has clearly pointed out that a society can only be humane if institutions do not harm the self-respect of citizens. Tronto (2013) points to the importance of the flexibility of institutions: "...when institutions are flexible enough to have several ways to meet people's needs, when no one acts out of neglect or abuse, then we will be able to say that we live in a caring society" (p. 164). Institutional hierarchies pose a threat to caring practices because the clarification and processes of practicing responsibilities is not ordered along the here and now demanding caring situations, but along abstract hierarchical positioning (Kohlen, 2014). Therefore, a move of ethics towards democratic care involves a flattening out of hierarchies.

STARTING THE PROJECT MOVING ETHICS

The director in charge of ethics of the PGD and the action researcher, author of this article, discussed how to start best by acknowledging the work that has already been accomplished by health care practitioners in the field of hospital ethics. We decided to design a questionnaire in order to see what has already been developed with regard to the typical tasks of HECs: education, policy making, and ethical case consultation. We decided to bring the questionnaire to the existing HECs in order to get to talk with the committee members about their current ethical concerns and activities before asking to fill in the questionnaire. The questions we wanted to have answers to were: "What are the ethics committee currently doing?," "Who are the leaders and members?," "What are the strengths and what are the weaknesses defined by committee members and others?," "Which rules have been worked on so far: communication, case-consultation models?," and "What can we conclude from the answers for the educational program?"

The following questions are the key ones that were asked in the questionnaire and asked during the visit to the committees: "Since when is your Ethics Committee working?," "What are your tasks?," "Which professions participate?," "Who is leading the committee?," "What are the competencies of the members?," "Do you have a working plan for this year?," "What kind of ethical education or training have you attended?," "What kind of education have you organized so far?," "Who is informed about your work?," "What kind of resources do you have?," and "What is important for you to bring your work forward?"

The answers revealed that the committees were in different stages of development. While some committees, either with or without being trained, started with ethical case consultation, others were just in the beginning of organizing their tasks. Thus, ethical case consultation—undertaken by members of the ethics committees—took place from none to 30 times per year in the hospitals. Ethics education had rarely taken place and none of the committees worked on policies. Some committee members (participants) were trying to define responsibilities for the committee work and had not identified leadership. Most of the participants who were questioned, talked about a *slow process* doing ethics and explained that professional support was needed. They complained that some kind of response to their ethical endeavors had not occurred. While a majority complained about structural deficiencies, some connected the deficiency to an erosion of their caring values. Some pointed out: "Of course, we care about patients' dignity and caring well, but we cannot see any structural support"; and "Where are the ethical values of the institution?" In sum, most of the participants expressed that the structural conditions were not beneficial to fulfill caring practices well, or *at all*.

From 2010 up to now, seven of the PGD hospitals are participating in the project, more services are joining in since 2014. Over the years, participatory research has shifted the emphasis from action and change to collaborative research activities. The joint process of knowledge-production has led to new insights on the part of both scientists and practitioners. As it is characteristic for participatory research the focus is on process, not on outcomes.

THE PARTICIPATORY ACTION RESEARCH PROCESS

Research strategies that emphasize participation are increasingly used in health research (Cornwall & Jewkes, 1995). Breaking the linear mold of conventional research, participatory research focuses on a process of sequential reflection and action, carried out with and by local people like health care practitioners rather than on them. Local knowledge like clinical knowledge, based on everyday practices and perspectives, are not only acknowledged but form the basis for research and planning. In conventional research and extension, inappropriate recommendations have frequently followed from a failure to take account of local experiences, priorities, processes, and perspectives. In contrast, in participatory research the emphasis is on a *bottom up* approach with a focus on locally defined priorities and local perspectives. Involving local people as participants in research and planning has been shown both to enhance effectiveness (Cornwall & Jewkes, 1995) and most probably save time and money in the long term.

In the project, Moving Ethics, the attentiveness to the practitioners' perceptions, the descriptions of their working realities, their problem definitions and ideas for solutions have been decisive for deciding to follow a collaborative participatory approach. Creating reflective spaces to identify and confront their problems has become not only essential as a primary step in the process of trust building and restoring confidence to engage in the collaborative process, but an ongoing recurrent element of the project.

It is not a question of creating a conflict-free space, but rather of ensuring that the conflicts that are revealed can be jointly discussed; that they can either be solved, or, at least accepted as different positions; and that a certain level of conflict tolerance is achieved. In order to facilitate sufficient openness, this space needs to be a "safe space" in which the participants can be confident that their utterances will not be used against them, and they will not suffer any disadvantages if they express critical or dissenting opinions (Bergold & Thomas, 2012).

PARALLEL: RESPONSIVE EVALUATION

Parallel to the action research, a responsive evaluation was carried out. In the action research, through a cyclic process of mutual learning, analysis, fact finding, planning, taking next steps, and evaluating, people are brought into the research as owners of their own knowledge, listen to different views and do empowerment to take action. Since the participatory approach aims at democratisation as a learning process of voluntary and responsible participation, a dialogical and responsive focused framework of evaluation was chosen for the project. Responsive evaluation is grounded in hermeneutic and constructivist perspectives of knowledge. In these perspectives, human beings are considered active interpreters of their world. The underlying ontological notion is that human beings are fundamentally relational. The meaning of the world is not given, but shaped in interactions and social relations. Meaning construction is a dialogical process (Greene & Abma, 2001; Stake & Abma, 2005). Epistemologically, these traditions are grounded in the notion that object and subject mutually influence each other (Abma & Widdershoven, 2008). Thus, the findings of a study are influenced by the interaction of the evaluator and stakeholders. Responsive evaluation has been conceptualized in different ways, from non-interactive to highly interactive. In the responsive approach to evaluation, as practiced in the project Moving Ethics, a maximum of inclusion and participation of stakeholders was allowed and energy invested into facilitating a dialogue among stakeholders in which differences in interpretation are respected and given meaning. "Differences in perspectives may lead to conflict among people and asymmetric power relations influence the way conflicts are handled" (Visse, Abma, & Widdershoven, 2015, p. 169). In case of a conflict, arising in the project Moving Ethics, a mutual work on keeping connected, respect different views and trying to understand each other was aimed at and a maximum of constructive communication involved. Conditions for the creation of spaces for resolving conflict (Tronto, 2010) were given by each of the three pillars of the model.

THE THREE PILLARS MODEL: EDUCATION, COMPANIONSHIP, AND OPEN SPACE

Along the participatory action research process, published experiences of actors in other hospitals organizing and doing clinical ethics (Krobath & Heller, 2010; Kobert, Pfäfflin, & Reiter-Theil, 2008) were brought in and discussed from a care ethical perspective. Experiences of success were reflected and questioned whether the underlying ideas of organizing and doing ethics would fit local conditions and resources (Kohlen, 2009b). The ideas were expanded on the basis of an analysis of local realities (Kohlen, 2015a). Care ethical questions about needs, attentiveness, responsibility, competence, and responsiveness (Tronto, 1993; Walker, 1998; Visse, 2016) as well as presence (Baart, 2010) were put forward and brought to a head by asking: In which way does this idea of organizing and doing ethics (not) contribute to be in touch with the patients, his and her families as well as professional actors in the field?

A threefold support for ethical work was developed and established from 2010 to 2012: (a) in relation to an ongoing ethical *education* and development of skills for and with committee members as well as for practitioners with an interest in clinical ethics; (b) in relation to *companionship* with a focus on team building and individual development of ethics committees; and (c) in relation to an *open space* to be informed about new ethical issues with relevance to clinical ethics, a discussion about what the information would mean for local activities, an exchange of experiences in each of the hospitals, and self-organization of collaborations. Thus, a three pillars model (Figure 6.1) emerged slowly and was explicated (Kohlen, 2015b).

Education

Education as one pillar of the model refers mostly to further educational classes about ethics consultation and takes place at the PGD Academy at Lutherstadt Wittenberg. The contents of the curriculum "Ethics Consultation in the Hospital" of the Academy of Medicine (AEM; Simon, May, & Neitzke, 2005) are met. The curriculum consists of three parts which can be put into three modules: (a) basics of ethics: theories, concepts, ethics, and the law; (b) the hospital as a learning organization: responsibilities and decision-making processes in the organization, models and structures of ethics

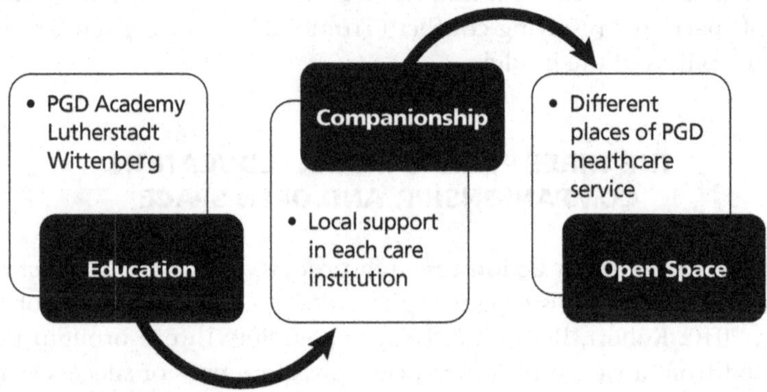

Figure 6.1 Three pillars model.

consultation, planning, and implementation, as well as evaluation of ethics consultation; and (c) consultation: aims and forms of consultation, tasks and methods, reflection of one's role and task, possibilities, and limitations (Simon, May, & Neitzke, 2005). The training of case consultation and trying out different methods takes plays in all modules. At the end of the training, each participant should be able to moderate ethical case consultations. A successful active participation of the three modules (Level 1) can be certified by the AEM. Participants who would like to work as a coordinator of clinical ethics can move on with ethics education (Level 2).

The ethics education at the PGD Academy Lutherstadt Wittenberg takes place at three different times over 1 year. Each module is taught within 2 days. In between the modules there is a phase of about 2 to 5 months to apply the ethical knowledge in practice, write about the experiences and bring them to class to be discussed. The exchanges of experiences and feedbacks are essential for a mutual learning process. Questions from the hospital arena and conflicts brought into class by participants, are attended to. A variety of learning methods, mostly scenery plays, are set into action for analysis, decision-making and problem-solving strategies (Scheller, 1998; Kohlen, 2003).

Companionship

The PGD ethics committees and working groups are individually supported in the development of their team—and ethics work. The support takes place in the different hospitals and integrates a reflection on local conditions and resources. At least every second year a whole day of coming together for reflection and next-year's planning is organized. What has been achieved in ethical work is reflected and evaluated. What should be achieved in the near future is planned and responsibilities who is going to do what till when with who are clarified. Especially in the beginning of implementing an ethics committee, the support is important with regard to organizational aspects and to secure that all standards of ethical consultation in health care institutions are met (AEM 2010, pp. 149–153). Moreover, trust building for successful team development is essential and needs careful attention within the second two years of implementation. Team development always needs special attention and can become a matter of concern when members (have to) leave the committee, get ill, or die. To make companionship work over years, the building of trust, bringing in plurality and learning to see and feel the values of communicating continuously in a respectful manner were essential and helped to prevent predicaments.

Open Space

The open space meetings aim at bringing solidarity alive among the different work of the PGD health care service and moving forward towards democratic care. Twice a year open space meetings take place for one afternoon (4 hours) by alternating the PGD locations: hospitals, nursing homes, or hospices. The aim of the meetings is to bring together all people of the PGD health care services who are actively involved in moving ethics as well as the ones who are interested in doing so. The meetings start with an opening hour to join into formal as well as informal talks by having drinks and finger food. Usually, the participants have just finished their work in the morning and they can use the opening hour as a break and a warming-up to get into ethical talk. The formal part of the meetings starts with reporting about the current state of moving ethics at PGD. After questions, discussions and an exchange of ideas, an ethics expert informs about new ethical issues and points to critical considerations. For example, the topics were: living wills, assisted suicide, advance care planning, and how to deal with dementia care in the hospital setting. A discussion follows and interest groups with a focus on special aspects and questions come together. The various groups discuss ideas about whether and how to put the presented ethical issue into action. Finally, the group ideas are brought together and written down by the moderation team. The ideas are discussed in the ethics committee meetings and refined for the individual hospitals. Support for implementation is given by the days of companionship and by further educational classes—offered at the PGD Academy—that focus on current ethical issues.

WHAT DID I LEARN? WHAT IS NEXT?

I was amazed about the deep commitment of the practitioners who want to move ethics by overcoming a strict hierarchy. Most of the committee members felt that they do not want to have a leader since this would not be fruitful for developing a shared-responsibility approach. The compromise: If, having a leader at all, it should be two leaders who share the responsibility in the organizing committee work. The pillar companionship turned out to be the perfect link between education and open space. What the practitioners learnt in class is applied and needs reflection in a team to overcome pitfalls and the illusion of fast progresses. A team that respects capabilities and competencies of its members needs to be developed. It is not just there. Doing companionship means getting to know what the real conflicts are and move to a clear analysis of what belongs to the field of ethics or needs to be discussed someplace else.

I have understood that highly structured approaches downplay the importance of dialogical interaction between the practitioners and the researcher. The more I structured the next step of the process the less creativity came up. Of course, I am not saying that structure is not necessary, but it is important to accept structures, at least sometimes, to be rather fluid in order to keep going with what is important as defined by the practitioners. I also learned that people in positions of power need to be involved in order to see what is going on, understand more about the ethics work, and what the effect of doing and moving ethics can be. Additionally, their involvement has to be real, not symbolic. The practitioners see and feel everything. If the people in positions of power do not bring their attentiveness and time to really get into a dialogue with the practitioners doing ethics and try to understand the conflicts due to structural constraints, there is the danger that their interest in a participation to move ethics is not taken seriously. Therefore, the researchers in the project need to point out the importance of the necessity of a real instead of a symbolic presence.

The whole action research project will be evaluated in depth in 2018. Instruments for evaluation are currently developed in cooperation with practitioners. Following the methodological premises of doing responsive evaluation, indicators and criteria for evaluation are determined by the stakeholders themselves. According to Robert Stake (1973), who developed the responsive approach, the issues and concerns of participants are the conceptual drivers of the evaluation process. The three pillars model will be compared to other models that were developed in other health care services, but which are not yet described.

KEY CONCEPTS

- moving ethics
- education
- companionship
- open space
- democratic care

DISCUSSION QUESTIONS

1. What would the three pillar model as proposed in this chapter, mean for the caring democracy that Tronto (2015) proposed in her book?
2. In what way was the responsive evaluation formative for moving ethics in this setting?
3. How does the three pillar model facilitate trust and solidarity, features of a caring society?

REFERENCES

Abma, T., & Widdershoven, G. (2008). Evaluation as social relation. *Evaluation, 14*(2), 209–225.

Baart, A. (2010). Die Kraft der Präsenz [The power of presence]. In H. Volker & M. Horstman (Eds.), *Wichern drei—gemeinwesendiakonische Impulse* [Wake up three-community-deaconous impulses] (pp. 142–150). Neukirchen-Vluyn, Germany: Neukirchener Theologie.

Bergold, J., & Thomas, S. (2012). Participatory research methods: A methodological approach in motion. *Historische Sozialforschung, 37*(4), 191–222.

Conradi, E. (2001). *Take care. Grundlagen einer Ethik der Achtsamkeit* [Take care. Basics of an ethics of attentiveness]. Frankfurt am Main: Campus.

Conradi, E., & Vosman, F. (Eds.). *Praxis der Achtsamkeit. Schlüsselbegriffe der Care-Ethik* [Praxis of Care. Key insights of care ethics]. Frankfurt am Main: Campus.

Cornwall, A., & Jewkes, R. (1995). What is participatory research? *Social Science Medicine, 41*(12), 1667–1676.

Greene, J. C., & Abma, T. A. (Eds.). (2001). Responsive evaluation: New directions for evaluation, No. 92. San Francisco, CA: Jossey-Bass.

Hart, E., & Bond, M. (1998). Action research for health and social care: A guide to practice. Buckingham, England: Open University Press.

Kobert, K., Pfäfflin, M., & Reiter-Theil, S. (2008). Der Klinische Ethikberatungsdienst im Evangelischen Krankenhaus Bielefeld. Hintergrund, Konzepte und Strategien zur Evaluation [Clinical Ethics Advisory Service in the Protestant Hospital Bielefeld. Background, concepts and evaluation strategies]. *Ethik in der Medizin, 20*, 122–133.

Kohlen, H. (2003). Ethikausbildung in der Pflege. Ethik im Kopf. Ethik vor Ort [Ethics education in nursing. Ethics in Mind. Ethics for Place.]. In C. Wiesemann et al. (Eds.), *Pflegeethik* [*Nursing Ethics*]. Stuttgart, Germany.

Kohlen, H. (2009a). *Conflicts of care: Hospital ethics committees in the USA and Germany.* Frankfurt, Germany: Campus.

Kohlen, H. (2009b). Wie sich ethische Konflikte (nicht) lösen lassen [How ethical conflicts can (not) be solved]. In G. Augustin, J. Reiter, M. Schulze (Eds.), *Christliches ethos und lebenskultur* [Christian ethos and life culture] (pp. 455–462). Paderborn, Germany: Bonifatius.

Kohlen, H. (2011). Care-Praxis und Gerechtigkeit. Der konkrete Andere in Medizin und Pflege [Care-Practice and justice. The concrete other in medicine and nursing]. In M. Dederich & M. Schnell (Eds.), *Können Anerkennung & Gerechtigkeit zu einer nichtexklusiven Ethik der Bildungs—und Heilberufe beitragen?* [Can recognition and justice contribute to a non-exclusive ethics for educational and health care professionals] (pp. 217–231). Bielefeld, Germany: Transcript.

Kohlen, H. (2014). If ethics in psychiatry is the answer—What was the question? Exploring social space and the role of clinical chaplaincy. *Aporia, 1*(14), 5–15.

Kohlen, H. (2015a). Ethik in der Organisation in Bewegung bringen—Überlegungen zu einer voraussetzungsvollen Idee [Bringing ethics in the organisation in motion—Thoughts about an that is based on requirements]. In M. Becka

(Ed.), *Ethik im Justizvollzug. Aufgaben, Chancen und Grenzen* [Ethics in prison. Tasks, chances and limits] (pp. 175–187). Stuttgart, Germany: Kohlhammer.

Kohlen, H. (2015b). *Klinische Ethik in Bewegung. Das Drei-Säulen-Modell Bildung, Beratung, Öffentlichkeit. Informationsbroschüre für die Paul Gerhardt Diakonie. Berlin* [Clinical ethics in motion. The three pillars model education, compagnionship, open space. An information brochure edited by the Paul Gerhardt Diaconia in Berlin].

Krobath, Th., Heller, A. (Eds.). (2010). *Ethik organisieren. Handbuch der Organisationsethik* [Organizing ethics. Handbook of organisational ethics]. Freiburg i. Breisgau: Lambertus.

Margalit, A. (1997). *Politik der würde* [Politics of dignity]. Berlin, Germany: Alexander Fest.

Scheller, I. (1998). *Szenisches spiel: Handbuch für die pädagogische praxis* [Scenary play. Handbook for educational praxis]. Berlin, Germany: Beltz.

Sevenhuijsen, S. (1996). *Oordelen met zorg: Feministische beschouwingen over recht, moral en politiek.* Amsterdam, Netherlands: Boom.

Sevenhuijsen, S. (1998). *Citizenship and the ethics of care: Feminist considerations on justice, morality, and politics.* London, England: Routledge.

Simon, A., May, A., & Neitzke, G. (2005). Curriculum "Ethikberatung im Krankenhaus." *Ethik in der Medizin, 4,* 322–326.

Stake, R. E. (1973, October). *Program Evaluation, in Particular Responsive Evaluation.* Paper presented at the new trends evaluation conference, Goteborg, Sweden.

Stake, R. E., & Abma, T. (2005). Responsive evaluation. In S. Mathison (Ed.), *Encyclopedia of evaluation* (pp. 376–379). Thousand Oaks, CA: SAGE.

Tronto, J. (1993). *Moral boundaries: A political argument for an ethics of care.* London, England: Routledge.

Tronto, J. (2010). Creating caring institutions: Politics, plurality, and purpose. *Ethics and Social Welfare, 4*(2), 158–171.

Tronto, J. (2013). *Caring democracy: Markets, equality, and justice.* New York, NY: NYU Press.

van Nistelrooij, I. (2014). *Sacrifice: A care ethical reappraisal of sacrifice and self-sacrifice.* Leuven, Belgium: Peeters.

Visse, M. (2016). Wessen Verantwortung? Auf dem Weg zu einem dialogischen Begriff [Whose responsibility? On the way to a dialogical notion]. In E. Conradi, & F. Vosman (Eds.), *Praxis der Achtsamkeit. Schlüsselbegriffe der Care-Ethik* [Praxis of attentiveness. Key concepts in care ethics] (pp. 209–231), Frankfurt, Germany: Campus.

Visse, M., Abma, T., & Widdershoven, G. (2015). Practising political care ethics: Can responsive evaluation foster democratic care? *Ethics and Social Welfare. 9*(2), 164–182.

Vorstand der Akademie für Ethik in der Medizin e.V. [Steering committee of the Academy of Medicine]. (2010). Standards für Ethikberatung des Gesundheitswesens [Standards for ethics consultation in health care]. *Ethik in der Medizin 22,* 149–153.

Walker, M. U. (1998). *Moral understandings: A feminist study in ethics.* New York, NY: Oxford University Press.

PART IV

RESPONSIVE EVALUATION FOR A CARING SOCIETY

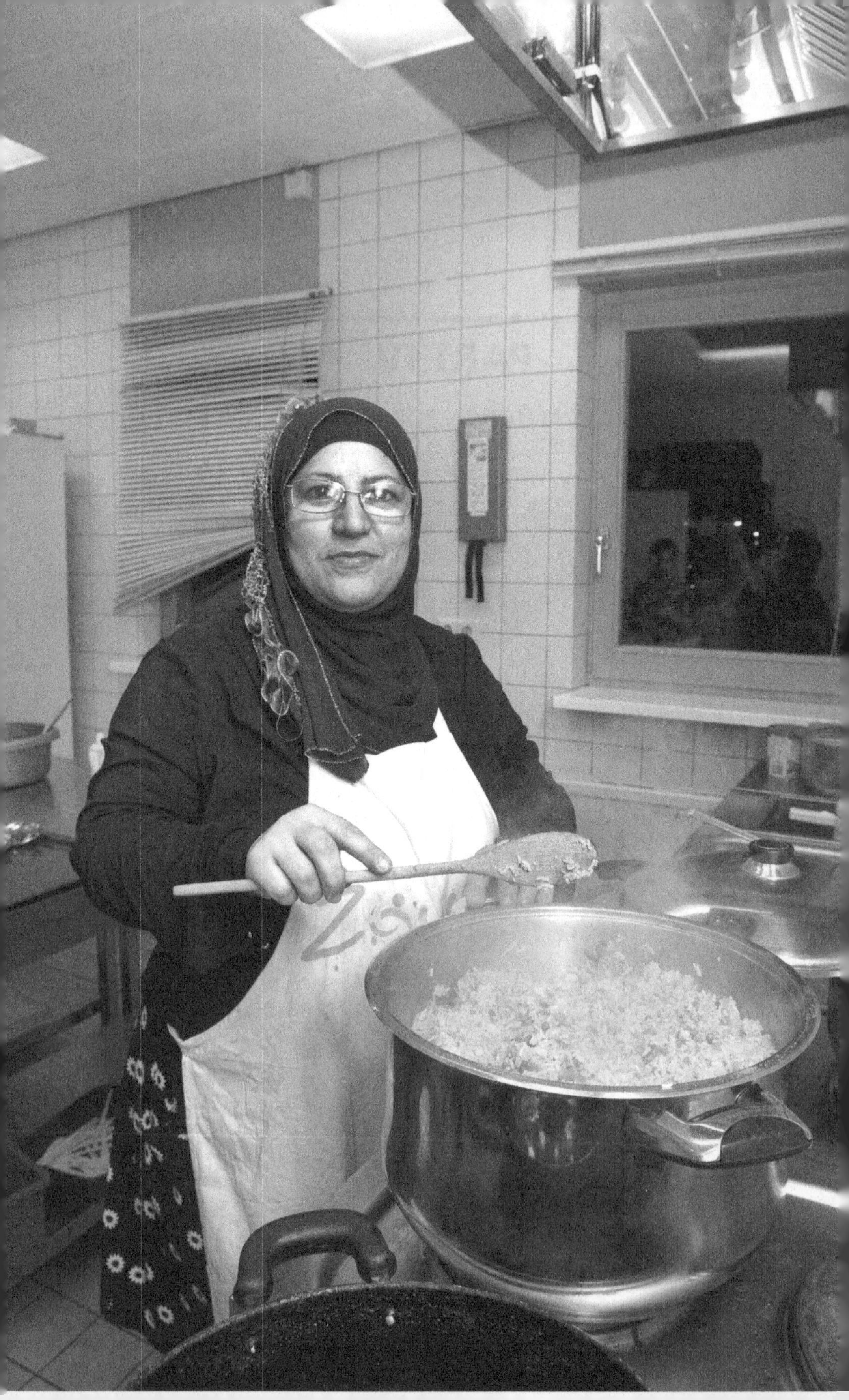

CHAPTER 7

RESPONDING TO OTHERNESS

The Need for Experimental-Relational Spaces

Gustaaf Bos and Tineke Abma
VU University Medical Centre/EMGO+

The history of people with a disability is one marked by being put aside, with labels such as impaired, defective, deviant, or abnormal (Goodey, 2011; Oliver, 1996; Ravaud & Stiker, 2001). Since the 1980s, as part of an emancipatory movement many people with disabilities have responded to this by raising their voice against the medical model that reduced them to their disability, and by protesting against stigmatizing labels, discrimination and marginalization. They have argued for a valued position in society, as full-fledged citizens (Atkinson, 1999; Goodley, 2011; Gray & Jackson, 2002; UPIAS, 1976), and lately policy makers worldwide have placed deinstitutionalization, normalization, inclusion, and participation on their agendas (United Nations, 2006).

Inclusion and participation policies aim to enhance the integration of people with disabilities in society. They range from dismantling large-scale institutions (Cummins & Lau, 2003; Mansell & Ericsson, 1996), through

Evaluation for a Caring Society, pages 159–183

widening the scope of exclusionary educational and vocational systems (Akkerman, 2016; EASNIE, 2016), to promoting and stimulating more space in the mainstream of our societies for the enriching facets of the full range of human diversity (United Nations, 2011).

In the Netherlands, a peculiar inclusion approach was developed, called *reversed integration* (Bos, 2016; Venema, Otten, & Vlaskamp, 2016). Reversed integration is a compromise between complete deinstitutionalization and maintaining large sheltered residential care facilities (Tweede Kamer, 1996). In reversed integration settings, people without intellectual or psychiatric disabilities move to an institutional terrain in order to live (or work or recreate) in the vicinity of the residents with intellectual or psychiatric disabilities. Policy makers believed that reversed integration could unite the better of two worlds: the freedom of movement, safety, and support services of a traditional residential care facility, and the everyday excitement and interactions of an ordinary neighborhood (Bos, 2016).

An underlying policy assumption was that people with said disabilities were more or less the same as people without a disability. Policy makers and advocate groups stressed that, although people with an intellectual disability might have less intellectual or cognitive skills, it was time to shift our attention and appreciation to the many commonalities between people with and without disabilities (Tweede Kamer, 1995). Thus, the policy focus was on fostering similarities and facilitating normalization. "Normalization" (Nirje, 1969), "social role valorization" (Wolfensberger, 1983), and the "citizenship paradigm" (Van Gennep, 1997) were considered as critical responses to an overly one-sided medicalized approach, which set people apart and focused on deviance. This preference for equality and equivalence appeared in many Dutch governmental and organizational policies and practices concerning the inclusion and participation of people with intellectual and psychiatric disabilities. It formed the basis of another related policy assumption, namely that the initial and new residents of reversed integration settings could interact meaningfully with each other and develop mutually rewarding relationships. It goes without saying that many embraced these policy ideals of inclusion and citizenship.

Yet, how people with severe intellectual and/or multiple disabilities—the initial residents of most reversed integration settings—could benefit from everyday neighborhood life remained unclear. Also, very little was known about how people without intellectual disabilities would actually respond to their neighbors with severe disabilities. Between 2010 and 2015, these knowledge gaps formed the background for a responsive evaluation (Abma, 2006; Abma & Widdershoven, 2014) in four reversed integration settings, which aimed to better understand and value what happened in encounters between the initial and the new neighbors. The idea was to set up dialogues among stakeholders, but soon the main evaluator, Gustaaf

Bos, began to realize that verbally mediated encounters were not particularly well suited to include people with severe intellectual disabilities. As he dearly wanted to include their perspectives, he felt the need to experiment with a more bodily, and a less verbal and cognitive approach and interpretation of such encounters.

The purpose of this chapter is to illustrate why it is both inescapable and crucial to strive for more experimental-relational spaces for differences between people with and without severe intellectual disabilities (or, people from the mainstream and people from the margins of our society). The main lesson we would like to share is that in our attempts to understand a "strange other" and to do right by him or her, we should try to attune bodily, modestly, acquiescent, trustfully, and reflectively to his or her otherness. We do so by presenting a story about encounters with Harry, one of the people that fascinated the evaluator. The story is interrupted by reflections from a care ethical perspective in the form of a dialogue between both authors. This text has the character of what Roland Barthes called a "writerly" text (Abma, 2002). A writerly text creates room for reflexivity and engages readers to think about and reinterpret/rewrite the text. It does not communicate a precise meaning or seek closure, and its openness fits well with the ethics of responsiveness, relationality and care we want to articulate in this chapter.

CONFUSING (AND UNSATISFACTORY) ENCOUNTERS WITH HARRY

Harry is one of the most fascinating characters I, Gustaaf (from now on I), have ever met. As a person with an intellectual disability he lived in one of the "reversed integration" settings. Harry—around 40 years of age—has a small, hunching posture and two remarkably blue eyes. In his neighborhood, Harry is well known for the way in which he frequently initiates physically intimate contact with people he meets on the street. After establishing eye contact, he tends to approach them rapidly with an excited smile on his face, grab their hand or arm and give them a long, piercing look from very close range. While doing so, he never speaks a word. Instead, he tends to moan, grunt, or make bark-like sounds.

The first time we met, I was utterly confused and alienated by Harry's candid advances. I felt a strong urge to push him back and walk away. After a couple of times, however, I realized that I foremost felt deeply unable to respond adequately to Harry. "Why did he approach me like this?," "What could he mean?," "What did he want from me?," moreover, "How was I supposed to communicate with him in a reciprocal way?"

Several of Harry's neighbors told me they shared similar feelings of disturbance and doubt in their encounters with Harry. According to two of them, Albert and Varela, the tendency to avoid this unpleasant sense of uncertainty led many neighbors to evade Harry in the street or to cut the encounters short.

> Albert: With some people it's impossible to connect. Harry, for example, [...] is someone who barely talks, but who can give others a deeply piercing look from a very close distance. Whenever he gets too intrusive, we simply say: "Harry, you'd better go to the community center." He always listens to that. But some people don't know how to handle him.
>
> Varela: The neighborhood kids do know this too. They also say, "Harry, you'd better go to the community center." And then he goes.
>
> (neighbors without intellectual disability, conversation report 870082, p. 3)

The overly physical and nonverbal way in which Harry expressed himself was so unfamiliar to me, that I was not only frightened but also fascinated by it. Was it really impossible to connect with him? In spite of my strong feelings of confusion and rejection, over the course of my fieldwork I repeatedly tried to interact more frequently and for longer periods with Harry, in order to get to know him better. However, without the means of sharing words, I continued to feel unable to communicate with him in a meaningful manner. As a result, our interactions remained rather brief, one minute at maximum. Each time, Harry seemed to lose interest in me quite rapidly, as I was struggling to connect and find out more about him.

Although my initial unease with the extraordinary bodily character of our encounters decreased over time, my confusion about the meaning of nonverbal encounters did not diminish at all. In the context of everyday neighborhood life, it seemed impossible to learn more about Harry's behavior, motives, issues, and values. After my first year of fieldwork, I did not even have a clue how to communicate with him in a meaningful way.

REFLECTION: HOW TO BE SELF-REFLEXIVE ABOUT YOUR OWN NEEDS AS AN EVALUATOR?

Tineke Wonders:

The mix of unease and value you endow to bodily experiences strikes me. I think—in line with care ethicists and Karin Dahlberg's chapter—that emotions are very important to deeply understand persons with intellectual disabilities and to value the encounters between neighbors. Special educationalist Max van Manen calls this *pathic knowing* (Van Manen & Li, 2002).

In care ethics, it is considered very important to pay attention to emotions. This is grounded in the notion that living a better life requires the embracing rather than "glossing over" of feelings. Glossing over feelings implies a superficial engagement with the emotional complexities of living practices such as those of caring and responsibility; what is required is a much deeper and emotionally challenging engagement that redefines our relationship with the world (Zembylas, Bozalek, & Shefer, 2014). This is what I see in your work. But what does this mean for you as a person and evaluator?

What about the unease and your own needs? Self-care is another important notion in care ethics. Caregivers such as teachers and others involved in hands-on caregiving processes—like you as responsive evaluator—can be so focused on the needs of others that they do not pay enough attention to making sure that their own needs are cared for. It is important to be self-reflexive about our own needs for care. Caring is a deeply emotional process that highlights the entanglement between reflection, emotion, and care of the self. How have you dealt with this, Gustaaf?

Gustaaf Responds:

You touch a deeply intriguing theme here.

Let me start by saying that I have a very strong urge to feel attached, connected to the people in my vicinity; I quickly feel miserable and unsafe if I do not feel noticed by them. Such a perceived lack of attention or recognition can easily make me feel utterly discouraged and inadequate.

All of this has to do with sharing time and positive attention, benevolence. The feeling that I am recognized and acknowledged. This attention is given in different ways, for instance by someone's willingness to respond to my questions, or because he or she smiles at me or touches me to show he or she somehow appreciates my presence. A sense of shared vicinity.

It also has to do with the "rush" of experiencing a shared understanding, or better yet: a shared pursuit of mutual understanding, wherein the will to search together is the unifier.

I have to admit that my thinking about this has not yet come to an end. Before my fieldwork, I used to think that my feeling connected to someone was primarily dependent on shared characteristics—hence I was often looking for those during encounters with others. However, through interacting with people like Harry I realized that contact without words frequently made me feel liberated for some time and free from my thoughts and judgments, my certainties and doubts. During these moments, I felt strongly connected with them, despite all the uncomfortable and confusing otherness I perceived. Experiencing such a thorough connectedness with people in whose company I usually perceived more differences than commonalities, in an unfamiliar (care) context and without the ability to apply my trusted verbal and rational communication device, often touched me deeply—and time and again urged me to new reflection processes (Bos, 2016).

Halfway during the second year, as my frustration about the seemingly nonsensical and superficial interactions with Harry in the neighborhood setting kept growing, I had the opportunity to spend more time around him: six consecutive days of participant observation in the neighborhood petting zoo where he participated in daytime activities. These 6 days in the petting zoo—a comforting, activating, and familiar environment, surrounded by people Harry was familiar with (his fellow clients, support staff, and a few regular visitors)—brought me an enriching and stimulating exchange of perspectives about him, myself, and possible ways for us to interact. In the following paragraph, after the reflection, I would like to share three examples of such learning experiences.

REFLECTION: HOW TO DEAL WITH YOUR PRIVILEGED POSITION AND (IR)RESPONSIBILITY?

Tineke Wonders:

What comes to mind is your own privileged position (and of mine also of course), of not being disabled. It is hard to imagine what it means to live with an intellectual disability; let alone to live with an intellectual disability in a world that circles around intellect, cognition, and high speed. In our Western culture, intellect and cognition are considered so important, they are the standard for normalcy.

How to deal with our privileges?

Care ethicist Joan Tronto (1993) has coined the notion of "privileged irresponsibility" referring to the way power and privilege works (p. 121). A privileged position allows one not to take care, to be irresponsible. To leave the caring work to others, migrants, people in lower positions, women. This is not to say that you behaved that way. But to a certain extent you were there in the position just to watch and observe, not to care.

Or did I miss something? Did you actually do caring work? Here I do not only refer to a disposition, being empathic and so forth, but to the labor of caring. Care ethicists point out that caring is a laborious activity which involves several aspects including thought, emotion, action, and work. Could you reflect on that, Gustaaf?

Gustaaf Responds:

At the very start of my PhD research, my formal role was acting as a participant observant in various residential care settings for people with intellectual disabilities. Rather soon I found out that in these care settings I was never the only one who decided about my role and position. What I could and could not do was largely determined by the demands and routines of the residents and the staff. Hence, in these residential care settings I was often pushed into a caring or supporting role.

Throughout my participant observations I thus performed several formal caring tasks, such as assisting people with eating and bathing, putting on people's coats, tying their shoelaces, and walking with people in wheelchairs. Besides, I spent many hours with the residents sitting, listening, chatting, drinking coffee, enjoying their music, and looking at their photos—care activities of which many professionals said they regretted that they hardly found time for in the hectic everyday.

Although I enjoyed the vast majority of these interactions, I kept feeling ambiguous about the (limited) ways in which I was allowed to perform in reversed integration settings. To what extent was my assisting residents with intellectual disabilities caused by a *care giver reflex*, a pre-reflexive tendency that is embraced by many people without disabilities once they interact with someone with disabilities, and a reflex that helps them to evade an imminent uncomfortable encounter? Was it not possible to interact in a more horizontal, human-to-human way with the original residents? Or were these preeminently examples of human-to-human interaction, containing norms with which I, as an outsider and an active member of our partly digitalized society, was hardly familiar with?

This ambiguity with regard to my role also entailed questions about which values constituted my privileged position compared to the original residents of reversed integration settings. I am aware that it might be perceived as perverse and unjust to complain about loss from a position of power (Young, 1997) and to idealize the position of the marginalized party (Waldenfels, 1990/2013), but still: From my academically encapsulated position, I frequently experienced a profound loss—a deep inability to relate adequately to persons like Harry, whom I had to consider as my participants.

THREE INSPIRING EXAMPLES

My first (and to me a most remarkable) observation was that no one in the petting zoo ever asked Harry to go someplace else, no matter how physically close he came. Instead, whenever he grabbed their hand or arm, leaned against them and stared intensely, the people present either greeted him kindly, made a joke-like comment, or asked him if everything was okay. Although he never responded verbally to such utterings, both Harry and the people he approached seemed to like interacting in this way: Throughout the week, he repeatedly approached them, and he kept receiving similar responses. Apart from these regular communicative initiatives, Harry mainly kept to himself and more often than not tended to withdraw to one of the sheds, or under the canteen table, in the bushes or behind the hen house. This observation made me realize that interactions may still be mutually fulfilling when the people involved use communicative means that are incompatible at first glance.

The second thing that triggered me, presented itself in the interactions between Harry and Gerald, the zookeeper. As one might expect, Gerald the zookeeper coordinated the activities in the petting zoo; at the start of the shifts as well as after the breaks he gave the support staff and their clients a short briefing. Furthermore, throughout the day, he regularly made sure everyone was okay and everything went according to plan. During these coordinating activities, the only person he never approached directly was Harry; I never heard him talking to him nor did I catch him even looking in Harry's direction. At first I thought of this as a sign that Gerald was hardly aware of Harry's presence, but soon I realized that this interpretation was inaccurate. Gerald proved to be very aware of Harry's presence, however, he approached him only indirectly and tried to involve him actively but not before he was sure that Harry was interested. In order to get his attention, Gerald frequently tended to introduce a more or less puzzling object in Harry's vicinity.

One day for example, Gerald stood in front of the hen house with a thick piece of rope and a pair of scissors. This performance caught the attention of Harry, who was crouching in the bushes behind the hen house. Apparently, Gerald was trying to cut off a piece of rope, but he had to make a real effort because the scissor blades were rather blunt. While struggling to cut the rope, he made eye contact with Harry. Then, without saying anything, he stretched his arms in Harry's direction, as to hand over the scissors and the rope. Harry jumped up, walked quickly in Gerald's direction, grabbed the scissors and tried to cut through the rope. He also struggled for a while, gave up, handed back the scissors, smiled briefly at Gerald and disappeared quickly behind the hen house again. "Almost," Gerald mumbled, and went on with his round.

Another time, when the zookeeper was talking to a visiting mother and child and Harry quietly tried to creep along, Gerald interrupted the mother to ask the child with an emphatic tone of voice: "Do you want a piece of candy?" Harry immediately froze and turned around, with an expectant look on his face. Gerald caught his eye and asked, quasi casually, "Do you also want a piece of candy, Harry?" Quickly, Harry approached the three with an enthusiastic grin. Gerald, the mother, and child looked at him and laughed. Then, the four of them went together into the zoo canteen to get something sweet.

From these interactions between Gerald and Harry I learned that it was possible to change roles in the interaction with Harry and to initiate longer lasting contact with him, by introducing something that interested him—not only *without* but also *with* words (at least he knew the meaning of the word candy).

The third interaction that struck me, took place inside the small petting zoo canteen, at lunchtime on the third day of my participant observation, between Harry and Adriane, his very agile and talkative 20-year-old co-worker with an intellectual disability.

> It is quite noisy in the small canteen. With eight people, all the seats are taken. While enjoying their sandwiches, most of the people present enjoy a lively group conversation. No one seems to pay attention to Harry, who hunches on a stool in the corner of the canteen. He seems nervous, his eyes go back and forth through the space and he rubs his hands. Although his open lunch box rests on his knees, he does not eat anything. Suddenly, Adriane walks up to him and gently puts her hand on his shoulder. Instantly, he starts staring at her, with a radiant and hopeful expression on his face. The hand rubbing intensifies. Then Adriane whispers to him, "Come on." Immediately, Harry stands up, takes Adriane's hand and huddles up to her. Adriane then puts her arm around his shoulders. In this intimate pose, they leave the canteen together, their lunch boxes in their hands. The other people present do not seem to have noticed anything out of the ordinary; the lively group conversation continues. After a while, I quietly follow Adriane and Harry outside. They are sitting close to each other beside the pond, some twenty meters away from the zoo, eating in silence. Occasionally, one of them throws a piece of bread towards the squawking ducks.
>
> (Fieldnotes, January 27, 2012, pp. 34–35)

Apparently, Adriane responded very adequately to Harry's nonverbal demand. She adapted her (predominantly verbal) communication style to his essentially nonverbal, bodily way of expressing himself, in order to take control over the situation and to communicate with him in a meaningful manner.

Later that day, Adriane gave me her assessment of the situation. In her opinion, Harry simply needed less excitement in order to get to his lunch. To her, that was all there was to it. However, I could not help but think that for this specific situation to alter, someone (i.e., Adriane) had to: (a) renounce her predominantly verbal communication style, (b) touch Harry's body, and (c) let her body be touched by his. Furthermore, it was not only by her sensitive attuning to his essentially bodily interaction style, but also by her directing and joining him to a quieter place, that Harry was able to come to peace and to enjoy a shared lunch.

REFLECTION: HOW TO REBALANCE POWER RELATIONS AND TO SHOW YOUR VULNERABILITY?

Tineke Appreciates:

What I especially like here is that you learn from a guy who is working in the zoo, and a person with intellectual disabilities. Here you turn around the hierarchy between social positions. Usually laborers (as opposed to people who use their heads) and people with intellectual disabilities are considered the ones who are lower in the hierarchy. They are often thought of as people who have difficulties with learning or cannot learn at all. Those without such disability are in the position to share their knowledge and intellect and teach those with a disability or with a lower educational background. You turn this around and convincingly show that we can learn from people with a lower educational training background and with intellectual disabilities. In fact, you portray them and show us that they are very wise, socially and emotionally developed, but also morally virtuous.

What I liked about the story of Adriane is that people with an intellectual disability are not only care receivers but also caregivers. This is commonly overlooked. People with a disability are primarily conceived as care receivers. This puts them in a position where they are framed as passive, dependent on others. Here, you show us that this frame is not correct. Care ethicists have also pointed out that all human beings are caregivers and receivers. So, thank you for illuminating this!

I wonder whether this rebalancing of power relations was something intentionally done, sought for? What was it like to show and face your own vulnerability?

Gustaaf Answers:

If our society validates the notion that we can hardly learn from people who did not receive (prestigious) formal education, then I fully reject this. After all, this misguided idea ignores the importance of implicit, tacit, bodily, and experiential knowledge, and of the wisdom of life. Besides, multiple contemporary scholars illustrate convincingly how fruitful a horizontal dialogue between academic, professional, and experiential knowledge can be, in terms of applicable policies and interventions (e.g., Weerman, 2016).

Nonetheless, during my fieldwork, I was repeatedly reminded of the hegemonic position that academic knowledge tends to hold in the contemporary care discourses. Many care professionals, family members, volunteers, and new residents treated me as if I, as an academic researcher, would know what was best when it came to encounters between people with and without intellectual disabilities ("You are one of the smart guys"). This prejudice was at odds with the dialogical character of the responsive methodology, the pursuit to produce shared knowledge in a horizontal way. It was due to moments like these, that I became extra aware of the impact of asymmetrical relations on the mental distance and the fragile relation of trust between the stakeholders of a responsive research project. And, consequently, on the knowledge which people felt safe to share or not.

All this urged me once more to take as much time as possible to get acquainted with the perspectives of the people involved, with special attention for those who were at the highest risk of being ignored, stigmatized or marginalized.

A GRADUALLY CHANGING PERSPECTIVE ON KNOWLEDGE PRODUCTION

The three aforementioned learning experiences inspired me to think about communicating with Harry in ways I had not tried before.

First of all, they made me realize that I, as an outsider, had falsely presumed that Harry, because of his clear preference for nonverbal communication, did not appreciate to be spoken to, did not understand the meaning other people attached to spoken words and was not able to attach meaning to verbal utterings himself. However, the three examples clearly show that the shared meaning making processes between Harry and the other participants were indeed partly verbal (i.e., joke-like comments, "candy" and "come on").

What remained unclear to me at that point was how Harry attached meanings to the words of others. To what extent were his responses based on the "what" of their messages, and to what extent the "how," on his relation with them and/or on the interaction context?

With this question in the back of my mind I experimented a little with verbal sense making in my interactions with Harry. On the fourth day of my participant observation, I asked him on two different occasions to do something with an object, deliberately without looking at the object and without suggesting gestures or mimicry. First, I asked him to throw a plastic cup in the trash bin of the canteen and later on, in the yard, I asked him to pick up some withered branches. Both times, Harry responded adequately to my demand, without any visible doubts. To me, from a social psychological and communicational point of view, this was a puzzling observation. If Harry—at least in the familiar context of the neighborhood petting zoo—was able to respond adequately to merely verbal, random communication acts of a relative stranger, why was it that in the majority of his everyday encounters with (familiar) others—both in the petting zoo and the neighborhood—he seemed not so much interested in what they said as well in how they looked and felt? What did Harry appreciate so much in the nonverbal, bodily and tactile aspects of his interactions with others that this made him seemingly negligent towards what they expressed with their words?

Recalling the three aforementioned examples, I realized that it was impossible to come any closer to appreciating why Harry interacted with other people in the way he did, if I did not reflect on what his communication partners expressed towards him (partly by means of words). Hence, I compared what I had been doing in my two short verbal experiments to how Gerald, Adriane, and the other people in the petting zoo responded to Harry. In what way did my responding to Harry's presence differ from theirs?

It appeared to me that the main difference was that I, as an evaluator, had tried to get to know Harry better by using my academic frame of reference. However, since this approach had not yielded any more insight into his perspective (or even constructed new knowledge), an obvious (and fundamental) step I had to take was to let go of my strong orientation on the verbal, cognitive, and rational aspects of communicating with Harry.

Doing this forced me to recognize that my discomfort and confusion about the bodily and nonverbal way in which Harry responded to other people (and me) appeared to be intertwined with my stubborn verbal attempts to attach cognitive, rational meanings to what happened in his encounters with others. This relational insight justified the question what I was actually doing with those words and cognitive frames of reference, whether or not inspired by social psychology or communication theory. Why did I keep using them so persistently, when they did not bring me any closer to understanding Harry?

A plausible answer is that I stayed so academically occupied in a futile attempt to gain more control over the interactions and the physical distance between Harry and myself. Put differently: I applied verbality and cognition as weaponry to defend and protect my own weaknesses. This metaphor makes sense, because all of my previous encounters with Harry confronted me with at least two of my vulnerable sides.

The first soft spot is that I find it generally unpleasant to be in someone's vicinity without being able to share words—especially if the other person is unfamiliar to me. Being able to exchange words gives me a feeling of control over the encounter: I can use my verbal input to influence the atmosphere and steer the interactional structure. When I find myself nearby someone without the possibility of verbal communication, I often feel rather inept and powerless; uncertain about how to behave and, consequently, strongly preferring to withdraw from the situation.

Secondly, a nonverbal encounter hampers my tendency to make things look better or to look at them from a different perspective. As a result, in nonverbal encounters I cannot take a certain distance from (potentially) overwhelming experiences or emotions. Without words and models no theories to interpret something and to gain more insight; no clear-cut opportunities for developing and expressing a new point of view. Consequently, everything I noticed between Harry and myself had an extremely unfiltered, intense and confusing impact (Bos, 2016, p. 99).

A SILENT (AND SATISFACTORY) ENCOUNTER WITH HARRY AND THE GOATS

Acting upon this relational insight to what seemed to be happening between Harry and me, on the last 2 days in the petting zoo I consciously tried to be less verbal and more receptive (or vulnerable) in our interactions. In other words: I intended to respond to him and follow him more intuitively, without the aim of catching him in one of my (academically nourished) frames of reference. To my excitement, this "open" attitude immediately and clearly changed the pattern in which Harry and I hitherto interacted with one another. This considerable change can best be illustrated by a completely wordless and 15 minutes (!) long encounter near the goats' pasture behind the petting zoo.

> While making some photos of the jumpy goats, I suddenly notice Harry in the middle of the pasture, some 30 meters ahead. He is running around between the goats, making yelp-like sounds. As soon as he sees me, he hurries in my direction. I keep looking at him. Harry runs towards the fence that surrounds the pasture and leniently climbs over it. He grunts and walks towards me, with an [expectant] expression on his face. I hold my tongue and look at him with a smile. With a grin from ear to ear, Harry grabs my arm and gives me one of his most piercing looks. I keep looking back at him with a smile. Like that, we stand in front of each other for at least two minutes.
>
> Although I feel a growing urge to say something—anything—I manage to keep silent.
>
> When I cannot stand the awkwardness of this situation any longer, I knock on the wooden bench beside us and sit down. Harry immediately sits down next to me, with an excited expression on his face. When I look silently into the pasture in front of us, my sight is almost blinded by the sharp beam of the low winter sun. I squeeze my eyes, enjoying the brightness. Looking beside me, I see that Harry is also squeezing his eyes in the sunlight. After a while, he looks back at me, smiling. I return a smile. When I look into the pasture again, he does the same. And when I look back at him again, he acts likewise. We keep exchanging gazes and smiles, without words or sounds.
>
> After a couple of minutes, Harry points towards two nosy goats near the fence in front of us. He winks at me, walks to the fence, and pets one of them. I follow him and pet the other goat. As soon as I do this, Harry looks at me with a euphoric smile. I smirk back at him, feeling deeply relieved and happy at the same time.
>
> When the two goats start frolicking again, Harry and I return to the little bench. We sit down to enjoy the bright sunshine, the playful goats and each other's company. In complete silence.
>
> (Fieldnotes, January 27, 2012, pp. 38–39)

REFLECTION: HOW TO PREVENT CARING PRACTICES IN BECOMING SUPERFICIAL AND SENTIMENTAL?

Tineke Comments:

In your account, Harry comes to life. We see and feel that Harry is better off in the petting zoo than in the care institution. The notion of human flourishing comes to mind, the ultimate goal of care ethics. Here I can see that you are also focused on human flourishing, and implicitly I also read that you are critical of the situation in which Harry is not reaching his full human potential. This reminds me of the notion that caring practices may be superficial and sentimental, if they do not challenge inequalities. What is your view on this? Why do you, for example, focus on inspiring examples? And what is inspiring for you? Does this resonate with the aspect of Tronto's caring definition that care involves repairing our world in order to live in it as well as possible? This incorporates a notion of human flourishing; care is thus seen as essential for human and environmental survival and flourishing.

Gustaaf Acknowledges, Confirms:

Without any doubt, I was determined to try to get to know Harry better. I wanted to find out who he was, what kept him going, what made him happy, and what he was concerned about.

Hence, I could not accept that Harry's (physical) attempts to get closer to his neighbors were best off with a response of sending him away, widening the gap. But what was a better option? Apparently, alternatives had to be found in the realm of unusual, atypical, not everyday interaction styles. But how so? Such was—and still is—the quest.

If you mean by me being "critical of the situation in which Harry is not reaching his full human potential," then you are absolutely right. The search for better, and more gratifying contact with Harry kept me, in the words of phenomenologist Bernhard Waldenfels (2010), "awake from the sleep of normalization" (n.p.). The frequent sending away of Harry by his neighbors, whenever he came too close (literally and figuratively), as well as the fact that he immediately obeyed them, unmistakably shows the skewed power relations between Harry and his new neighbors. It also illustrates the large extent of communicative inflexibility and social clumsiness from Western, modern, individualized, and increasingly digitalized communities concerning everyday contact in public space.

Initially, this was primarily my own (professionally and personally motivated) quest, absolutely. I wanted my contact with Harry to flourish, because I presumed that this would help me flourish, and I hoped that this would also be the case for Harry. In that sense, my search was at least as much about the way in which I tried to reach my own full human potential in this situation—a potential that I deemed closely related to Harry's. Thus, a human potential that has a vast social foundation.

I agree with your suggestion that this search became more socially critical along the way. After all, I put my observations and reflections about encounters with Harry on paper, to take a stand against the asymmetrical dynamics and excluding mechanisms that dominate and order the seemingly self-evident ways in which many interactions between neighbors (and other people) with and without intellectual disabilities take place. My primary motivation for this is not so much the care ethical pursuit to "repair our world," as well as to present an appealing micro-level alternative, by which stakeholders without intellectual disabilities are given a possibility to reflect on their own share in the non-existing or flagging encounters with people with intellectual disabilities. I do this in the hope, that such processes of reflection on interaction dynamics and morals will facilitate change in local practices. Which might be seen as an attempt to repair a micro-world.

LESSONS FROM THE CASE WHILE THINKING WITH (CARE) ETHICAL THEORIES

Communicating with, and observing encounters between, initial and new neighbors as well as reflecting on his own experiences by means of autoethnography and by thinking with (care) ethical theories (Jackson & Mazzei, 2013), Gustaaf began to revaluate the notion of difference in inclusion and participation policies and practices. He discovered the value of bodily and emotional experiences and of *pathic* knowledge (Van Manen & Li, 2002), in interacting with and caring for people with an intellectual disability (Bos, 2016).

The Need for Experimental-Relational Spaces of Encounter

Based on this insight, we argue that there is a need to work on more *experimental-relational spaces* be it work-, leisure-, neighborhood-, community-, or care-related—for encounters between marginalized people and people from the mainstream of our society to happen.

Such spaces of encounter are experimental, because beforehand none of the potential participants will know exactly, or know at all, what will happen, other than that strictly nonverbal encounters most likely will confront and confuse them—for the difference we will perceive is not by definition beautiful and enriching, but might also be frightening, eerie and difficult. Thus, encountering people in the margins of our society involves certain risks, or adventures, that people from the mainstream need to be willing to accept.

In order to accomplish this, the experimental spaces we advocate for necessarily have a relational character. Their starting point is the acknowledgment that any confused, fascinated, and/or evading response to the perception of the otherness of another person inevitably refers to ourselves in relation to this person: no one is ever strange on his own (Bos & Kal, 2016; Meininger, 2008; Waldenfels, 1990/2013). Recognizing this relational character of perceived strangeness in interactions with unfamiliar and marginalized others is crucial, because this very insight might inspire an interpersonal quest for more spaces for such encounters. From a care ethical perspective, we can see that in the story of Harry and Gustaaf the spark of energy between them began to flow when Gustaaf was opening himself by becoming aware of his own vulnerability. Through a reflexive stance, Gustaaf learned he had to give up his verbal weaponry and control over the situation—his privilege—in order to get to know and appreciate how to spend more time with Harry. This rebalancing of power created a situation for mutuality, where both were giving and receiving affectionate attention, and this created a feeling of mutual belonging. Indirectly, this implies a critical stance towards an overly cognitive, verbal, and rational society wherein people like Harry need to "fit in," and adjust themselves.

Heterotopia as Critical Relational Spaces for Encounters With Otherness

Ethicist Herman Meininger (2013) convincingly demonstrates that the Foucauldian concept of *heterotopia* is relevant in this respect. According to Foucault (1984; Foucault & Miskowiec, 1986), heterotopia (i.e., "other places" or "places of otherness") are counter-sites which reflect, question, and undo the logic of the *homotopia* (i.e., "normal places") of a disciplined society.

Meininger (2013) points out that traditional examples of heterotopia are prisons, psychiatric hospitals, and residential institutions for people with intellectual disabilities. These *total institutions* might be seen as symptoms of a society that strives to exclude all kinds of deviance (Foucault, 2006; Goffman, 1961). However, and paradoxically, from an ethical perspective, the people who are silenced and distanced from the heterotopia maintain powerful positions in the societal margins. They do so by being "others," by occupying the spaces that normality has abandoned—spaces, which continuously criticize, liquidate, or reverse "the self-propelling power of the othering and excluding normality" (Meininger, 2013, p. 28).

In line with Foucault (1984; Foucault & Miskowiec, 1986), Meininger (2013) shows that it is of utmost importance to recognize that, although some of the traditional (physical) forms of heterotopia still exist today, in our times space increasingly takes the form of relations among sites (i.e., is no longer demarcated by visible borders).

The reversed integration settings offer a good example. Typical total institutions open their territory to neighbors and people from the mainstream to create possibilities for interactions with people with an intellectual disability. The resulting deterritorialized interhuman connections are all but neutral and symmetrical, as we have seen in the story of Harry and his neighbors: Harry was sent away whenever he started puzzling interactions; the new neighbors were in control. Through a heterotopic lens, reserved integration settings are social spaces that create a complex power dynamics between people labelled as "intellectually disabled" and those in homotopic positions of power: legal representatives, physicians, psychologists, service providers, neighbors, family members, and so on (Carlson, 2010, in Meininger, 2013, p. 28). Hence, what we can refer to as *the homotopia of contemporary society* are monologic communities and communication styles which are dominated by what is meaningful and manageable to legal representatives, physicians, psychologists, service providers, neighbors, and family members. On the other side of the homotopic coin we see an evasion and exclusion of relations and interactions, which seem irrelevant and intangible for the powers to be—although these might be meaningful and manageable for people with intellectual disabilities.

Consequently, the heterotopia of our times—counter-sites that critically reflect, neutralize or invert the aforementioned societal focus on equality and equivalence—are no longer concrete geographical spaces on the margins of "normal" society, but consist in connections between people who live on the margins and people who live in the mainstream of civil society (Villadsen & Wyller, 2009). In other words: contemporary heterotopia are relational spaces of encounter, where people who are "other" to each other meet and communicate (Meininger, 2010, 2013).

Therewith, heterotopic spaces are distinguished from homotopia by their devotion to dialogue between the normal and the abnormal, order and disorder, the familiar and the strange. Essential thereby is how one participates in these dialogues and "whether one is being confronted, touched, and changed" (i.e., othered) by them (Villadsen & Wyller, 2009, as cited in Meininger, 2013, p. 32).

Unknowable Otherness Demands Moral Humility and a Passible Performance

Closely related to Meininger's work, the responsive ethics of phenomenologist Bernhard Waldenfels (2010) holds that, if we try to understand another person, we must recognize that his or her otherness is fundamentally unknowable to us. After all, for physical reasons as well as due to differences in life history, social position, experiences, and habits, it is impossible to take someone else's standpoint, to see and feel the world as he or she does (Waldenfels, 2004, 2011). Or, as political philosopher Iris Marion Young

(1997) puts it: If we strive for a democratic dialogue, we must acknowledge the *asymmetrical reciprocity* that inevitably influences this very dialogue.

According to Waldenfels (2010), recognizing the indisputable brokenness of our efforts to get to know the other, forces us into an ongoing rethinking and reflection. Hence, the insufficiency we experience when trying to do right by another person is the driving force behind a permanent searching, responsive-ethical attitude; a sting that keeps waking us from *the sleep of normalization* (cf. Irigaray, 1974; Meininger, 2007; Young, 1997).

In this regard, Young (1997) writes about the importance of "moral humility" (p. 350). From a morally humble starting point, we acknowledge that is impossible to see the world through the eyes of another person, but we are determined to gain more insight into the extent in which we share comparable experiences. Young claims that we probably will listen more sensitively to individual-specific expressions of personal experiences, interests, and claims, if we keep in mind that there will always be aspects of our communication partner and his or her situation that we will not understand. Moral humility in a dialogue with people from the margins of our society that bears a strong resemblance to what philosopher Jean-Francois Lyotard (1983/1988) coined as a "passible performance" (p. 168): the pursuit to keep listening in a sincere manner and to postpone any kind of interpretation or judgement—despite our experiencing of reflexive tensions—based on a desire to remain uncertain (for the time being; Brons, 2014). According to philosopher and activist Doortje Kal, the primary target of passibility is "to uncover the pretentious, apparently closed and definite character of 'normal' practices as being premature and not tenable. The current norms are temporarily suspended, in order to find out whether or not they need a transformation or supplement" (Bos & Kal, 2016, p. 131; cf. Kal, 2001).

In line with the previous, the experimental-relational spaces of encounter we advocate for, are defined by a searching, wondering and open-minded perseverance towards people who appear strange to us, intertwined with a determination not to colonize, socialize or tame their otherness with images which are more familiar to us. Hence, precisely the inerasable differences between people from the mainstream and people from the margins of our society ought to be the starting point for us to think about and work towards more spaces for horizontal interactions. The core of these relational spaces of encounter might be in staying with the other despite not knowing exactly, or not knowing at all, what he or she means; for instance through humor, smiling, playfulness, attentive watching, listening, touching and sensing, and without (too many) words (Bos & Kal, 2016).

A sincere, humble and passible way of responding to otherness may teach us many surprising and confusing things, not *just* about people with severe intellectual and/or multiple disabilities, their life worlds and the ways in which they shape their life in interactions with others (Goode, 1994), but always about ourselves in relation to them (Meininger, 2008; Waldenfels, 2011).

EXTENDING RESPONSIVE METHODOLOGY

The aforementioned encounters between the evaluator and Harry shed light on some of the limits of the responsive methodology; or rather—more generally—the borders of what counts as social scientific practice. The evaluator had to cross these verbal and cognitive borders, pass the Habermassian notion of dialogue as the verbal interchange of rational arguments. He had to conceive dialogue as both interaction and motion, whereby participants respond to each other, each other's position and each other's particularity—by means of their language, bodies, attitudes, and/or emotions (Bos, 2016; Niessen, 2007). From this stance, dialogue is seen as a *dia-logos* (literally: between logics) with an *intercorporal* character: the "how" and the "what" of any encounter moves among different logics and happens between and because of the bodies of the participants (Ntourou, 2007 in Meininger, 2013; Waldenfels, 2004). Ergo: When we desire to understand someone else, we need not only attend to words but to everything that happens between us. In the same vein, we are not only concerned about the content of the utterings of our communication partner, but also about their relation to us and to the context of our interaction (Watzlawick, Beavin, & Jackson, 1967/2011).

In the case in question, a responsive research approach aiming for horizontal (verbal) dialogue did not bring us any closer to the perspective of Harry. It rather produced knowledge about the evaluator in relation to Harry's particular stance in the world, and about possible ways in which the evaluator could interact with this otherness without quelling it.

Because the evaluator nevertheless tried all he could to gain more insight into the perspective of people like Harry, he was in continuous motion; thinking, doubting, and hesitant about the nature and the meanings of the own and the alien, the familiar and the unknown. This uncertain quest was confusing and tiring, exhausting at times. At certain moments, the evaluator desperately applied academic frames of reference or care professionals' jargon to attach meaning to, and gain control over, this uneasy otherness. Still, he kept struggling with these hegemonic and impersonal perspectives, since he wanted to try to do right by the perspective of Harry—although with time he realized that succeeding would be partial at best. Harry's otherness remained unknowable and unidentifiable for him—and thus all the responses the evaluator would offer to this otherness would inevitably fall short, wrench, and scrape.

Although seemingly inadequate at first glance, we think that such a searching, doubtful attitude is at any time preferable for social scientists to holding on to an all-embracing, homotopic perspective that claims otherness as a knowable variant of normality (whether exotic or not), or tries to render it as unobtrusive as possible (Bos, 2016).

In our view, the discussed case poses responsive methodologists the challenging question whether they—in their pursuit for more social equality and justice—are able to create space for nonverbal, noncognitive and nonrational ways to encounter their respondents, and consequently, assemble and produce interactional knowledge that aims to do justice to the perspectives of people who cannot speak for themselves.

REFLECTION: IS EVALUATION CARING WORK?

Tineke Asks:

We are working and exploring the crossroads between evaluation and caring. I think that your work as evaluator can be defined as caring work if we follow the definition of care as put forward by Berenice Fisher and Joan Tronto in 1991 (pp. 40–41) and later repeated in Tronto's seminal work entitled *Moral Boundaries* (1993, p. 130). They defined caring as follows:

> On the most general level, we suggest caring be viewed as a species activity that includes everything that we do to maintain, continue, and repair our "world" so that we can live in it as well as possible. That world includes our bodies, our selves, and our environment, all of which we seek to interweave in a complex, life-sustaining web. (Fisher & Tronto, 1991, pp. 40–41)

I think many evaluators do not consider their work as a form of caring. Caring is usually considered as the work done to help the sick, the weak, and the poor. We have had lengthy discussions on this topic with other evaluators and other authors of this book. So, for me it is important to know how you envision this. Do you agree and also feel in retrospect that what you did, that your evaluative work was in fact caring?

Reflection of Gustaaf:

Thank you for the interesting parallel you offer between caring and doing responsive research in a care setting. I agree that there is quite some overlap between the two, a thought that I would like to substantiate by specifying the definition of care.

To me—and I follow ethicist Herman Meininger (2002) here—caring for people with intellectual disabilities has everything to do with a trustful intention to encounter the other, based on the belief that it is possible to get to know him better. This susceptible, wondering, and passible attitude (Brons, 2014) is embedded in an everyday ethics of care. According to ethicist Hans Reinders (2000), this everyday ethics of care enables care professionals to create and develop moral qualities in the search to do right by the people they care for. In order to do justice, caregivers need to develop relational perspectives on (the life worlds of) the people they care for: lively, attracting, and/or prickly images, which are inevitably connected with their own view of man and worldview. These images are neither neutral nor fixed; they are rather ongoing and open to dialogue (Meininger, 2002). Because such a relational definition of caring is embedded in everyday ethics, it can only be found within the activities of the caregivers: in their trying to relate in the most adequate way to the other. Therefore, it is crucial for caregivers to acknowledge the asymmetrical power relations between professionals and clients. Thus, they should always keep trying not to fill the shoes of the people they care for, and be aware that they do not dominate them (Reinders, 2000; see Bourdieu, 1982, 1989).

In my view, the aforementioned description applies not only to professional caring acts, but also to the acts of evaluators of care practices. Both care professionals and responsive evaluators need to be willing to engage in relational acts of caring, in order to get to know the people they interact with better, and to be able to try to do right by their perspectives.

ACKNOWLEDGMENTS

The authors wish to thank Herman Meininger and Doortje Kal for their valuable comments on an earlier version of this text, and Audrey Wijnberg for carefully editing our English.

KEY CONCEPTS

- responsive evaluation
- experimental-relational space
- bodily knowing/learning
- bodily encounter
- writerly text
- power
- vulnerability
- prickly (unknowable) otherness
- responsive ethics
- moral humility
- nonverbal dialogue

DISCUSSION QUESTIONS

1. How can evaluators create space for nonverbal, noncognitive, and nonrational ways to encounter their respondents?
2. This chapter highlighted the importance of more bodily (and less verbal and cognitive) approaches and interpretation of encounters between people from the mainstream and people from the margins of our society. This is closely related to what Maurice Hamington asserted in chapter 1 when he writes that competent care engages both generalized knowledge, as well as concrete knowledge, the knowledge of the particular individual to be cared for. How does the view of Bos & Abma relate to Hamington's thoughts on to these kinds of knowing?
3. As this chapter has illustrated, this writerly text (Abma, 2002) creates room for reflexivity. It does not communicate a precise meaning or seek closure, and its openness fits well with the ethics of responsiveness, relationality and care. How would this way of writing fit in your own scholarly work?

REFERENCES

Abma, T. A. (2002). Emerging narrative forms of knowledge representation in the health sciences: Two texts in a postmodern context. *Qualitative Health Research, 12*(1), 5–27.

Abma, T. A. (2006). The practice and politics of responsive evaluation. *American Journal of Evaluation, 27*(1), 31–43.

Abma, T. A., & Widdershoven, G. A. M. (2014). Dialogical ethics and responsive evaluation as a framework for patient participation. *The American Journal of Bioetics, 14*(6), 27–29.

Akkerman, A. (2016). *Job satisfaction of people with intellectual disabilities: Associations with job characteristics, fulfilment of basic psychological needs and autonomous motivation* (Doctoral Thesis). VU University, Amsterdam, Netherlands.

Atkinson, D. (1999). *Advocacy: A review.* Brighton, England: Pavilion.

Bos, G.F. (2016). *Antwoorden op andersheid. Over ontmoetingen tussen mensen met en zonder verstandelijke beperking in omgekeerde-integratiesettingen* [Responding to otherness: About encounters between people with and without intellectual disabilities in 'reversed integration' settings] (Doctoral Thesis). VU University, Amsterdam, Netherlands.

Bos, G. F., & Kal, D. (2016). The value of inequality. *Social Inclusion, 4*(4), 129–139. doi:http://dx.doi.org/10.17645/si.v4i4.689.

Bourdieu, P. (1982). *La sociologie de Bourdieu.* Bordeaux, France: Mascaret.

Bourdieu, P. (1989). *Opstellen over smaak, habitus en het veldbegrip.* [Essays on taste, habitus and the field concept]. Amsterdam, Netherlands: Van Gennep.

Brons, R. (2014). Waardenwerk voor de strijdigheid van het bestaan. [Virtuous work for the contravenity of life]. *Waardenwerk, 57,* 72–84.

Cummins, R. A., & Lau, A. L. D. (2003). Community integration or community exposure? A review and discussion in relation to people with an intellectual disability. *Journal of Applied Research in Intellectual Disabilities, 16,* 145–157.

EASNIE. (2016). *Raising the achievement of all learners in Inclusive Education. Literature Review.* Odense, Denmark: European Agency for Special Needs and Inclusive Education.

Fisher, B., & Tronto, J. C. (1991). Towards a feminist theory of care. In E. Abel, & M. Nelson (Eds.), *Circles of care: Work and identity in women's lives* (pp. 36–54). Albany: State University of New York Press.

Foucault, M. (1984). Des espaces autres [Of other spaces]. *AMCS, Revue d'architecture,* (Octobre), 46–49.

Foucault, M. (2006). *History of madness.* Abingdon, England: Routledge.

Foucault, M., & Miskowiec, J. (1986). Of other spaces. *Diacritics, 16*(1), 22–27.

Goffman, E. (1961). *Asylums: Essays on the social situation of mental patients and other inmates.* Garden City, NY: Anchor Books.

Goode, D. (1994). *A world without words: The social construction of children born deaf and blind.* Philadelphia, PA: Temple University Press.

Goodey, C. F. (2011). *A history of intelligence and "Intellectual disability": The shaping of psychology in early modern Europe.* Farnham, England: Ashgate.

Goodley, D. (2011). *Disability studies: An interdisciplinary introduction.* London, England: SAGE Publications Ltd.

Gray, B., & Jackson, R. (2002). *Advocacy & Learning Disability.* London, England: Jessica Kingsley.

Irigaray, L. (1974). *Speculum of the other woman* (Gillian C. Gill, Trans.). Ithaca, NY: Cornell University Press.

Jackson, A. Y., & Mazzei L. A. (2013). Plugging one text into another: Thinking with theory in qualitative research. *Qualitative Inquiry, 19*(4), 261–271.

Kal, D. (2001). *Kwartiermaken. Werken aan ruimte voor mensen met een psychiatrische achtergrond* ['Setting up camp': Preparing a welcome for people with a psychiatric background]. Amsterdam, Netherlands: Boom.

Lyotard, J. F. (1988). *The differend: Phrases in dispute.* Minneapolis, MN: University of Minnesota Press.

Mansell, J., & Ericsson, K. (Eds.). (1996). *Deinstitutionalization and Community Living. Intellectual disability services in Scandinavia, Britain and the USA.* London, England: Chapman and Hall.

Meininger, H. P. (2002). *Zorgen met zin. Ethische beschouwingen over zorg voor mensen met een verstandelijke handicap* [Meaningful caring: Ethical reflections on care for people with an intellectual disability]. Amsterdam, Netherlands: SWP.

Meininger, H. P. (2007). Verbindende verhalen en de ruimte van de ontmoeting [Connective stories and the space of encounter]. In H. P. Meininger (Ed.), *Plaatsen waar plek is* (pp. 19–32). Amersfoort, Netherlands: 's Heeren Loo.

Meininger, H. P. (2008). The order of disturbance: Theological reflections on strangeness and strangers, and the inclusion of person with intellectual disabilities in faith communities. *Journal of Religion, Disability & Health, 12*(4), 347–364.

Meininger, H. P. (2010). Connecting stories: A narrative approach of social inclusion of persons with intellectual disability. *ALTER, European Journal of Disability Research, 4*(3), 190–202.

Meininger, H. P. (2013). Inclusion as heterotopia: Spaces of encounter between people with and without intellectual disability. *Journal of Social Inclusion, 4*(1), 24–44. Retrieved from https://josi.journals.griffith.edu.au/index.php/inclusion/article/view/252.

Niessen, T. J. H. (2007). *Emerging epistemologies: Making sense of teaching practice* (Dissertation). Fontys Hogeschool: Maastricht, Netherlands.

Nirje, B. (1969). The normalization principle and its human management implications. In R. Kugel & W. Wolfensberger (Eds.), *Changing patterns in residential services for the mentally retarded* (pp. 19–23). Washington, DC: President's Committee on Mental Retardation.

Oliver, M. (1996). *Understanding disability: From theory to practice.* Basingstoke, England: Macmillan.

Ravaud, J. F., & Stiker, H. J. (2001). Inclusion/Exclusion: An analysis of historical and cultural meanings. In G. L. Albrecht, K. D. Seelman, & M. Bury (Eds.), *Handbook of Disability Studies* (pp. 490–512). Thousand Oaks, CA: SAGE.

Reinders, J. S. (2000). *Ethiek in de zorg voor mensen met een verstandelijke handicap* [Ethics in the care for people with an intellectual disability]. Amsterdam, Netherlands: Boom.

Tronto, J. C. (1993). *Moral boundaries. A political argument for an Ethic of Care.* New York, NY: Routledge.

Tweede Kamer. (1995). *De perken te buiten: Meerjarenprogramma intersectoraal gehandicaptenbeleid 1995–1998* (No. 24170, nrs. 1–2) [Passing the bounds: Multiannual programme intersectoral disability policy 1995–1998]. The Hague, Netherlands: Sdu Uitgeverij.

Tweede Kamer. (1996). *Actualisatie 1996: Meerjarenprogramma intersectoraal gehandicaptenbeleid 1995–1998 De perken te buiten* (No. 24170, nr. 16) [Update 1996: Multiannual programme intersectoral disability policy 1995–1998 Passing the bounds]. The Hague, Netherlands: Sdu Uitgeverij.

United Nations. (2006). *Convention on the rights of persons with disabilities and optional protocol.* Washington, DC: United Nations.

United Nations. (2011). *Best Practices for including person with disabilities in all aspects of development efforts.* Washington, DC: United Nations Department of Economic and Social Affairs. Retrieved from http://www.un.org/disabilities/documents/best_practices_publication_2011.pdf.

UPIAS. (1976). *Fundamental principles of disability.* London, England: Union of the Physically Impaired Against Segregation.

Van Gennep, A. T. G. (1997). Paradigmaverschuiving in de visie op zorg voor mensen met een verstandelijke handicap. [Paradigm shift in the vision on care for people with an intellectual disability]. *Tijdschrift voor Orthopedagogiek, 36,* 189–201.

Van Manen, M., & Li, S. (2002). The pathic principle of pedagogical language. *Teaching and Teacher Education, 18,* 215–224.

Venema, E., Otten, S., & Vlaskamp, C. (2016). Direct support professionals and reversed integration of people with intellectual disabilities: Impact of attitudes, perceived social norms, and meta-evaluations. *Journal of Policy and Practice in Intellectual Disabilities, 13*(1), 41–49.

Villadsen, K., & Wyller, T. (2009). From the spatial heterotopos to the deterritorialized (heterotopic) hope. In T. Wyller (Ed.), *Heterotopic citizen. New research on religious work for the disadvantaged* (pp. 218–229). Göttingen, Germany: Vandenhoeck & Ruprecht.

Waldenfels, B. (1990/2013). *Der Stachel des Fremden* [The sting of the alien]. Frankfurt am Main: Suhrkamp.

Waldenfels, B. (2004). Bodily experience between selfhood and otherness. *Phenomenology and the Cognitive Sciences, 3,* 235–248.

Waldenfels, B. (2010). Response and trust: Some aspects of responsive ethics. New York, NY: Stony Brook State University. Retrieved from https://www.youtube.com/watch?v=t6iOsQ_ho94.

Waldenfels, B. (2011). In place of the other. *Continental Philosophy Review, 44,* 151–164.

Watzlawick, P., Beavin, J. H., & Jackson, D. D. (1967/2011). *Pragmatics of human communication: A study of interactional patterns, pathologies and paradoxes.* New York, NY: W. W. Norton and Company.

Weerman, A. (2016). Ervaringsdeskundige zorg—en dienstverleners. Stigma, verslaving en existentiele transformatie [Social workers with experiential knowledge: Stigma, addiction and existential transformation]. Delft, Netherlands: Eburon.

Wolfensberger, W. (1983). Social role valorization: A proposed new term for the principle of normalization. *Mental Retardation, 21*(6), 234–239.

Young, I. M. (1997). Asymmetrical reciprocity: On moral respect, wonder, and enlarged thought. *Constellations, 3*(3), 340–363.

Zembylas, M., Bozalek, V., & Shefer, T. (2014). Tronto's notion of privileged irresponsibility and the reconceptualisation of care: Implications for critical pedagogies of emotion in higher education. *Gender and Education, 26*(3), 200–214. doi: 10.1080/09540253.2014.901718.

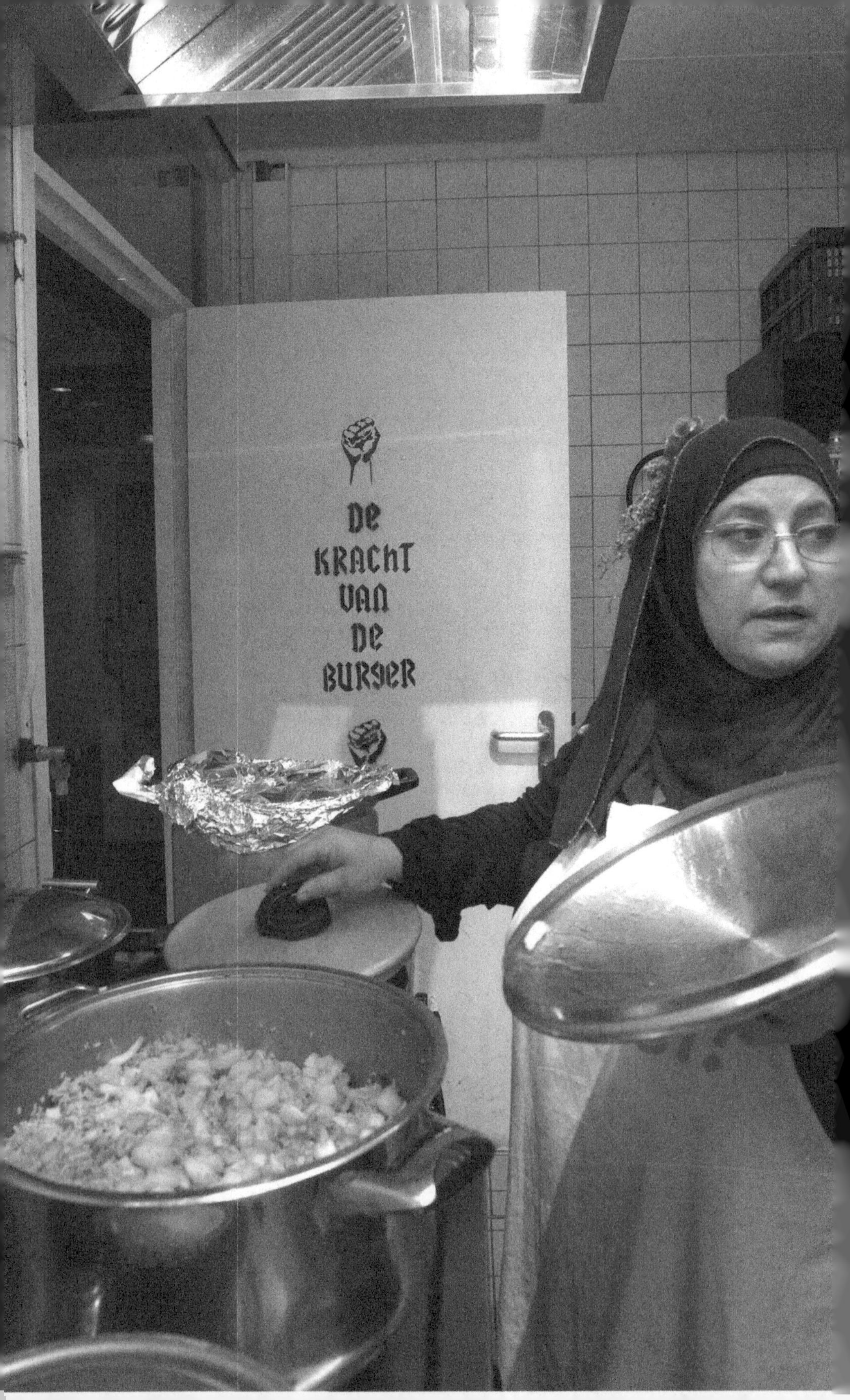
DE
KRACHT
VAN
DE
BURGER

CHAPTER 8

DIALOGUE, DIFFERENCE, AND CARE IN RESPONSIVE ENACTMENTS OF A WORLD-BECOMING

Melissa Freeman
The University of Georgia

This was our first meeting with the Young Docents' Club[1] (YDC), a museum-based, academic program for African-American teens in the Northeast. There were nine teens: four boys at one end of the long table and five girls at the other. Gail, the educational coordinator and former YDC coordinator was there, as well as Cynda, the brand new YDC coordinator. I was there, along with classmates from a course on participatory evaluation, to learn to conduct an evaluation by doing one. Since there were six of us forming the evaluation team, we scattered ourselves around the table so as not to form an obvious "them and us" division. Cynda suggested we all introduce ourselves, which we did. She then said we could do better than that and why don't we go around again and this time make a rhyme with our names. The girl next to her was asked to start but was unable to think of anything. Cynda

Evaluation for a Caring Society, pages 185–204

suggested a rhyme, which brought some snickers and some not so very nice other suggestions mumbled by other teens. At that point Gail spoke up and in a controlling manner asked us to explain the evaluation process to the teens and what we wanted from them. Without acknowledging Cynda's attempt to break the ice, we complied with Gail's demands and explained the interactive, responsive, and formative nature of our process and the desire to get to know the teens better. We suggested pairing each of us up with two teens, but also invited other suggestions. This led to some tentative suggestions, with some preferring to take a group approach, while others expressed being comfortable with being paired up. Gail suggested we come to the teens' weekly counseling session which sent ripples of resistance among the teens, which, in turn, prompted Gail to accuse us of not providing the teens enough structure. We repeated our desire to get to know the teens better as the beginning point for establishing a direction for the evaluation and that deciding between pairing up or establishing some sort of group process couldn't be that difficult.

Suddenly many people were talking at once, recirculating the concern for the lack of structure or offering ideas about the choices. At this point I felt that I was functioning (or not functioning) at many levels. At one level I felt trapped. I didn't know whether to contradict the members of my evaluation team, those who kept making statements confirming our lack of structure and those who were beginning to add to Gail's lecturing tone towards the teens. On another level, I was also sucked into the process with no clue as to how to escape from it. I had no idea what I was or was not "allowed" to do, as if there was some sort of convention of collaboration that should have been established to guide me. And at a third level, I was increasingly annoyed. Why was Gail so upset with us offering choices to the teens—How much more structure did she expect? So when someone suggested we split up—meaning the evaluators should step outside for a moment—I was just happy to get away even though it felt wrong to begin a participatory evaluation project in such a way.

After 15 minutes, Cynda sought us out and told us calmly that the teens needed a few ice breakers, but then would be glad to be paired up with us individually. Then Gail came over and, uptight and accusing, told us that we were not talking to the teens at their appropriate level of development. Teens couldn't function in an open conversation and needed structure. I reminded her that we had offered them a concrete choice and asked her how one could make it more structured, at which point she said we needed to tell the teens what we wanted, not give them a choice. We went back to the table with no better idea of how to "tell" the teens that we wanted to get to know them, and simply restated the two options while also reminding them that participation is always voluntary and not obligatory.

At that point the hawks who had gathered descended upon us. It was obvious that they did not like that voluntary business at all. For some reason, other museum staff had shown up and all of them were hovering over the teens and us. We were given a very disempowering lecture about how much this evaluation means to the museum and that helping the museum helps the teens. This was disturbing although very exciting. One staff member was saying that they needed more time to talk and prepare the teens before the evaluation begins, while I kept thinking, "I have been evaluating all along!" Nevertheless, this lecture was not right, especially for Cynda and the teens. Gail had basically taken the control right out of their hands and we had been incapable of providing a means of helping them take part in the process. Cynda's style is warm, encouraging, although she is nervous and the teens don't know her well. Gail, on the other hand, was directive saying things like: "David, have you been paying attention?" or "That is an inappropriate way of answering" to another. And yet it was Gail who had told us that the teens were familiar and comfortable with an open-ended process and Cynda who had expressed feelings of concern that the process might be overwhelming.

The message, however, for us (including the teens) to hear was clear. We had failed. The evaluation team and the teens could not be trusted to know what to do. Instead of providing more space for us to get acquainted, we were smothered and shut off. How are we going to break out of that? How can we establish rapport with the teens and the museum staff in such a context? Whose perspective on the teens was more accurate? While I had clear biases and believed not only in open-ended dialogue but in teens' capacities to engage in such dialogue, I was also reading Lisa Delpit's 1988 essay, "The Silenced Dialogue." In this work, she cautioned educators to think more critically about the way our processes, even those intended to include diverse perspectives, were not only filled with hidden assumptions about others, but could be silencing and disempowering to the very others we were hoping to include. Fortunately, even though I was white, our evaluation team was diverse. Hopefully, as a group, we could find a way to engage in a dialogue that would enable us to learn from each other, as well as from the museum staff and the teens.

This journal entry was written almost 20 years ago but it still reflects many of my values and concerns. More knowledgeable perhaps and more experienced conducting evaluations in diverse cultural and educational settings, I am still unsure how best to make use of dialogue in formative, responsive evaluations. Dialogue, to me, best represents the movement, purpose, and ethical values of responsive evaluation, and yet I find myself questioning, not its utility, but its conceptualization. This paper then serves as a turning point in my thinking about the role and meaning of dialogue in evaluation. To do this, I make several conceptual moves. First, I rethink my encounter at the museum not in regards to the success or failure of the dialogical encounter but as an enactment of responsiveness and relational ethics. From an ethics of care perspective, dialogue enables a diverse group of stakeholders "to be recognized as active participants in care" (Visse, Abma, & Widdershoven, 2015, p. 2). Interactions, such as the one recounted at the museum, make visible the way care—care for self, care for others, care for a cause, care for the process, and the like—infiltrates all dialogical events, and, as such, this manifestation needs to be understood and accounted for when seeking to understand and reconceptualize dialogue.

I then turn to the issue of difference itself. Like other responsive evaluators, respect for difference and the important role different perspectives play in the development of deeper social understandings have underscored the work that I do. In his book, *Achieving Our Humanity*, philosopher Emmanuel Eze (2001) critically analyzes the role race and racism has played in philosophical developments in metaphysics and theories of rationality and morality. His account makes clear that, whether or not race and racial differences are considered to be real or constructed, the concept of race has been an active participant in the construction of the world, both physical and conceptual, and continues to disperse its effects in real, and often damaging, ways. Eze's work helps me stay focused on respect for difference as a guiding principle for evaluation, while also opening up questions about the locus of cross-cultural understanding and how such understandings could ever be achieved. Dialogue, as a potential and hopeful site for "dialogue across difference" (Burbules & Rice, 1991; Wadsworth, 2001), holds a place of virtue for individuals invested in social and political change (Richardson, 2003), a place of virtue that has been repeatedly criticized for standing outside and above the political-situational realities of human relating, and for requiring a certain kind of wisdom or competence for productive and genuine engagement (Kohn, 2000).

It is here that I would like to consider the ethical value of taking a posthumanist turn for responsive evaluation. A posthumanist perspective does not eliminate or blur distinctions between humans and nonhumans, males or females, blacks or whites, but seeks, instead, to understand how such distinctions come-into-being in everyday practices. The point here is that much is missed in our attempts to understand difference when we assume that such things as humans, nonhumans, culture, race, care, dialogue, or wisdom exist prior to their being "differentially constituted" in the materializing practices of becoming so differentiated (Barad, 2007). Rather than assume predetermined differences between individuals, Karen Barad's (2007) agential realism helps us understand that inquiry must account for how differences are continuously being produced and performed. For example, the opening vignette could be read differently as an encounter where boundary markers such as "age," "race," "competence," "authority," and the like, are materialized in my account, whether intentionally or not, to denote, account for, and/or explain differences between our team's process and the expectations of the museum staff in regards to the youth.

Therefore, a final move that I make in my shift in thinking, is to draw on Barad's (2003, 2007, 2011) agential realism as a way to rethink dialogue as part of a posthumanist "ethics of entanglement" where entanglement is understood as "relations of obligation" (Barad, 2011, p. 150). An ethics of entanglement does not presume a best or right response to an "other" who stands before us, but orients itself toward "responsibility and accountability for the lively relationalities of becoming of which we are a part" (Barad, 2007, p. 393).

I will argue that while responsive evaluation has effectively put us in the midst of things, and has made visible the issues and diverse interests involved in particular settings, responsive evaluators have struggled with how to account for and work with this diversity. Furthermore, evaluation as responsiveness towards others "as others" unwittingly opens up a space where evaluation becomes complicit in the construction of a particular kind of diversity that positions individuals and groups at odds with each other, as holding different conceptions of reality, and as caring for different outcomes. What motivated my posthumanist turn is that I do not believe that any one person or group of people hold authority over what matters or have fixed and unified beliefs about what matters. When we predetermine that certain concepts, such as *authority* or *care* are possessed by some humans and not others, rather than consider that all entities—physical, discursive, or conceptual—become human, authority, or care when materialized as such within performed webs of relations, we prevent these human and nonhuman entities from materializing or being materialized in unexpected ways. Care, for example, as one such nonhuman entity, "is already operating in the space between agents" (Hamington, 2014, p. 198) and will manifest itself in the midst of our performance as caring agents. So trying to figure out what it *is* works against our ability to understand how it is performing. Looking back at the opening vignette, my journal entry suggests that what mattered to me at the time was our successful performance as an evaluation team. The entry reads as a series of failures—failure to build rapport, to gain trust, establish credibility, and so forth. Furthermore, in this account I turn to others, humans and texts, as experienced knowers to help me find my way in future encounters. Posthumanism does not discount these practices, or ask us to eliminate them. However it prompts us to turn our analytic attention away from these beliefs as predetermined markers of good practices for relationship building and seek instead to focus on how they, and other boundary-markers, have found themselves becoming stabilized as such. This way of thinking helps us examine "the practices through which these differential boundaries are stabilized and destabilized" (Barad,

2003, p. 808) in the performance of difference. It supports responsiveness and responsibility but in radically posthumanist ways.

RESPONSIVE EVALUATION AS RELATIONAL PRAXIS

Institutions can be formal or informal, physical or conceptual, emergent or imposed, but a characteristic they have in common is that they are manifestations of norms, beliefs, and traditions that organize social action and interaction. While some institutions are built to serve a specific group of individuals, others, such as public schools, must respond to the diversity of interests asserted by multicultural communities. Evaluation as the practice of forming a judgment about the worth, quality, or value of a program, object, individual, product, or institution plays a central role in constructing what a society considers significant/insignificant, normal/abnormal, or central/marginal. As such, it can play a crucial role in determining the nature and effectiveness of an institution's response to a diverse community. Because responsiveness is inherently relational, any evaluation approach seeking to understand or measure an institution's responsiveness must itself articulate a position on responsiveness and relationality.

Bob Stake's (1975) responsive evaluation has played a leading role in articulating a relational and responsive approach for evaluating programs and institutions. Rejecting the assumption that we can know what matters to stakeholders regarding a program prior to conducting an evaluation, responsive evaluation has provided an issue-oriented alternative. Stake (1975) explains: "Responsive evaluation is an alternative, an old alternative, based on what people do naturally to evaluate things, they observe and react" (p. 14). Crucial to his understanding is that when people react to something it is because that something is not sitting well with them; in other words, that *something* raises a question for them, prompting a stance of inquiry towards the activity or practice in question. Different people will react to different aspects of a program and these different issues and expectations are not only respected for the diversity of values they make visible, they are recirculated back throughout the course of the evaluation as conversations, draft reports, presentations, mock debates, and the like, as a way to prompt more responses and reactions. This dialogical process makes visible the complex range of stakeholder experiences and perceptions so they can fuel attention to deep-seated substantive issues, the kind that emanate from the root values that make us who we are and guide our way of being in the world. In other words, responsive evaluation makes understanding *praxis* its guiding principle. Unlike approaches guided by predetermined aims such as measuring program outcomes, responsive evaluation builds off of the activities and issues that make up practical life. Therefore, a focus on praxis as "the self-creative activity through which we make the world" (Lather, 1991, p. 11) supports the aim of responsive evaluation which is to provide a rich portrayal of the strengths, limitations, benefits, and harms of a particular program or institution and the ongoing appreciations, concerns, and desires of its constituents. The hope is that a program or institution will use this information to rethink, recreate, renew, or reject particular practices in ways that are constructively responsive to those most affected.

Evaluation and many other disciplines that are oriented to the practical "deal with ethical and political life; their *telos* is practical wisdom and knowledge" (Carr & Kemmis, 1986, p. 32). Educator Mark Smith (1994) explains that for Aristotle, praxis was "guided by a moral disposition to act truly and rightly, a concern to further human well-being and the good life. This is what the Greeks called *phronēsis,* and requires an understanding of other people" (p. 164). Phronesis is an important concept because it places judgment in the context of living rather than something that can be called upon and imposed on a situation like an external set of rules. Experience, discernment of hidden facets of a situation, and wisdom become important aspects of phronesis. This is because practical issues arise out of everyday situations. They are not planned in advance. As a result people must consider them in the context of a particular problem or situation and must respond to these based on what they consider to be good, useful, or beneficial to those involved. As such, responsive evaluation is also a "relational practice" (Visse, Abma, & Widdershoven, 2015, p. 6) guided by an ethics of care in that it consists of "interdependent human beings who need each other to understand and express who they are and what they think should be done in particular situations" (Visse, Abma, & Widdershoven, 2015, p. 4). Its intent is to surface or make visible confirming and conflicting positions on particular issues. A commitment to value pluralism guides the process.

By taking a posthumanist turn and attending to the activity of "worlding" (Barad, 2007, p. 160), or the way difference comes into being, I argue that evaluation can assist the ongoing task of redefining the role and place of institutions in a diverse society. A focus on worlding reorients responsive evaluation from being a practice that is responsive to diverse human interests, to one that is responsive to the world's ongoing enactment and reenactment of matter and meaning. Within this perspective, institutions are just one form these potential enactments might take, and are manifestations of the constitution of ethical life, as matter and meaning collide, intersect, and emerge in myriad ways. To transform ethical life, we must first understand it as inseparable to who we are as humans-in-the-world (Schmidt, 2012; Gadamer, 1989). To transform responsiveness we must no longer think of care as primarily that which prompts us to take action to enhance the well-being of ourselves or others (although this form of care is not unimportant), but as the visible manifestation of human and nonhuman relationality; care, uncaring, and carelessness, are all manifestations of complex values as these are enacted in the course of everyday "intra-actions" (Barad, 2007).

Responsive and other forms of evaluation create "an ethical space—that is, a space defined by a temporary suspension of normal ethical assumptions" (Kushner, 2000, p. 151). More importantly, Saville Kushner explains how evaluation as a practice establishes its own "moral order to which participants are expected to conform" (p. 152). This *moral order of, and by, design* is one I wish to consider in the remainder of this paper.

FROM RESPECT FOR DIFFERENCE TO ACCOUNTING FOR DIFFERENTIATION

The belief that others have something to teach me has held a central place in my approach to evaluation. As such my moral order has centered on respect for difference, attentiveness to making a space for value pluralism, and a deep commitment to dialogue as a necessary partner to praxis. To transform the world requires novel perspectives, visions, and ways of thinking that stretch the norm and go beyond what I alone can imagine. To understand what needs changing requires the sharing of successes, challenges, tragedies, and desires that I and others have lived, encountered, experienced, and overcome in a variety of ways. The surfacing of perspectives is only a first step, however, since developing a good understanding of core issues responsively is an iterative process that requires a certain kind of collective engagement. Crafting ethical spaces for collective engagement—critical, reflective, participatory, dialogical, or however conceived—must accomplish at least two things. It must be recognizable as a valid form of engagement by those who participate in it, and it must create a generative process whereby the varying perspectives on particular issues begin to foster new understandings that go beyond any one person's or group's values or beliefs without, at the same time, ignoring or discounting these values or beliefs. Dialogue, as characterized by Hans-Georg Gadamer has been conceptualized as having this potential. Philosopher Nicholas Davey (2013) explains that Gadamer's dialogical approach "implies that the mutual recognition that each party has different but supplementary interests in the truth of a subject-matter establishes the basis of a 'commonwealth' of mutually supplementing interpretations" (p. 109). Mutual recognition, Gadamer (1989) explains, "in a dialogue is not merely a matter of putting oneself forward and successfully asserting one's point of view, but being transformed into a communion in which we do not remain what we were" (p. 371). A genuine dialogue—that is, a dialogue that results in a giving over of oneself to the opportunity to have one's understanding transformed by opening up the multiplicities inherent in an issue is difficult to achieve. Gadamer's dialogical approach places ethical action in the midst of practical issues, as something emergent, not as something requiring knowledge of abstract theories or rules of conduct (George, 2014). However, dialogue itself as relational rides "on the concern to enact manners of being that are appropriately responsive to each context we find ourselves in, as well as on the cultivation of our ability thus to involve ourselves responsively" (George, 2014, p. 112). This cultivation, therefore, becomes an issue that needs to be addressed.

When I think of cultivation in relation to the context of the opening vignette, I am faced with a complex ethical dilemma. No matter how I think of cultivation in the context of the museum interaction (e.g., providing a roadmap to the dialogical process, establishing rules of respectful communication, building skills for dialogue, and so on), I am faced with needing to make preconceived assumptions about the "others" involved, whether those others are the youth, counselors, museum administrators, or my evaluation teammates. If dialogue is conceived of as something humans do, and something humans must learn to do well and respectfully as they share concerns, inquire into, and examine different perspectives on a topic that matters, then everything from the success of the interaction to the understandings generated rides on the capacities of those involved. What often ends up happening, as evident in the vignette, is that the focus becomes on *who* is participating in the dialogue and how those "whos" are performing, rather than on the issues that matter. What might my response have been if I had focused my journal entry on other entities? On the way our voices swirled together and collided, bringing concepts into being around the issue of "getting to know the teens"? Or on the various intentions and aims lurking behind our being there to conduct an evaluation? What "manner of questions regarding the nature of mattering" (Barad, 2012, p. 77) came together in this encounter?

Focusing on who says what and who is silenced puts emphasis on how the *who* is performing rather than on the performance itself. When dialogue, or other commonly used tools of engagement, is understood as something that mediates our understanding of self and other, it brings with it predetermined assumptions about these "selves" and "others" in relation to their capacities to perform this dialogical encounter together. This assessment can, and does, occur even when we understand the important role served by the inclusion of diverse perspectives in conversation. Gadamer (2000) explains this role:

> To allow the Other to be valid against oneself... is not only to recognize in principle the limitation of one's own framework, but is also to allow one to go beyond one's own possibilities, precisely in a dialogical, communicative, hermeneutic process. (p. 284)

Our tendency as humans who believe we have something important to say is that we often work against this potential and fail to preserve "the otherness of the other" as required for hermeneutic conversation (Schmidt, 2000, p. 360), and "reduce the other to the same" (Levinas, 1991, p. 43), and, in doing so, assume, or impose even, a predetermined "moral order" of appropriate conduct. A close analysis of the opening vignette clearly reveals aspects of the moral order that I expected of others in such a situation.

Diversity carries immanent risk. It makes visible alternative ways of being and knowing and as such threatens our social and cultural norms, our ways of acting and interacting, and what we believe to be right and good. Less well understood is how the markers of difference we have come to rely on to differentiate ourselves from others do not just indicate relativistic differences in social and cultural makeup but have seeped into our ways of seeing and thinking about who we believe should and could be doing the seeing and thinking. As Eze (2001) explains: "Questions about reason and human identity, including racial identity, have always clung together in modern thought, so that the dialectical movements of thought which organize the world, including our racial consciousness, present race to us as itself a domain of the rational" (p. 41). In other words, race and other identity markers are always, already present in our conceptualizations of the world. Furthermore, the very characteristics that make up a diverse people are used, on the one hand, to justify the oppression, silencing, marginalization, exploitation, persecution, and extermination of people not like ourselves, while, on the other, are employed as a source of pride, solidarity, empowerment, and epistemic privilege (Gilpin, 2006) as a way to overcome and resist oppression and exploitation. This makes "difference" a complex player needing to be included in any conversation on matters of importance. The question is what should this kind of inclusion look like? Why move beyond a conceptualization of dialogue as respect for difference to one of accounting for differentiation?

It seems clear that no matter how we conceptualize difference, the reality of its effects will always be with us, dividing the world up in particular ways. Seeking a future, therefore, where identity markers circulate in ways beneficial to those involved will require continuous attentiveness and anti-oppressive strategies. Eze (2001) writes:

> It is for us sufficient to indicate as postracial those moments, in thought and practice, where we acknowledge and work to overcome the explicit and the implicit racial social mechanisms operating to thwart opportunities for some and enhance opportunities for others. (p. 223)

Posthumanism, with its focus on explicit and implicit mechanisms for worlding, can become one of those anti-oppressive strategies. This requires a move beyond identity politics, not in the sense of discounting the way identity markers, such as race, gender, ability, sexual orientation, and the like, are used to create and/or resist divisions and distinctions between groups of people, but to seek out and recognize the way difference is produced, and make visible its disabling and enabling effects. This is a relational matter as educator Sharon Todd (2009) writes: "Pluralism is not simply about social attributes or identities; pluralism is also an indelible aspect of the emergence of subjectivity itself as a being-with-others" (p. 51).

A care ethics guided by posthumanism helps us see that care is not about responding to particular individuals or groups as if they stand for or embody some stabilized system of identification, but is a form of engagement that seeks to make visible the apparatuses that produce these differences. Again, the intent is not to eliminate difference, but to make visible and better understand the politics inherent in the design of who we are as people together. It asks us to reject the assumption of any one of us having predefined unique identities as we find ourselves responding to issues that matter. This rejection also includes predetermining the locus and nature of care itself. Therefore, I must amend Joan Tronto's (2013) statement that care, as a *human* expression, "always expresses an action or a disposition, a reaching out to something" (Tronto, 2013, p. x). Care is intra-active: carer, cared-about, being cared for all "come to matter, in the very terms of the encounter" (Johns-Putra, 2013, p. 129). Theorizing care as something that emanates from a *someone,* risks a dispersion of effects that takes us farther away from that which matters, rather than closer. The assumption of a *carer* creates certain dispositions that then stand outside and over the being doing the work. In other words, certain actions become labeled as "caring," are understood to be carried out by a "caring" person, which then assumes that other actions are not the result of "caring" or that there are "uncaring" people. Labels such as these, even ones with good intentions, result in divisions and the construction of false differences that are often no longer connected to the action itself. So, while I have always thought of evaluation as human expressions of care, I must move away from the idea of "care as a theory regarding the conscious development of self and citizenship" (Hamington, 2014, p. 204) in search of an understanding of care as an intra-active agent in its own right (Johns-Putra, 2013).

From a posthumanist perspective, dialogue and care perform along with other entities, whether human or nonhuman in a perpetual movement of becoming that gets differentiated as "human," "care," or some other notion that matters in that particular situation. "Understanding care as *performative* means understanding that our well-being and the well-being of all beings is indivisible. Thus care for and by 'the environment' is care for 'life in general' as it un-differentially cares for the life of humans" (Fry, 2011, p. 207, emphasis in original). In other words, care performs with other participating entities as they intra-act in the materializing practice we call *life* or *evaluation.* In such a practice, "subject, object, world and worlding all turn in relation to each other in that relational play of design(ing) that ontological design names and enacts" (Fry, 2011, p. 206). Although Tony Fry is talking about sustainability, I find his idea of design having its own agency intriguing. In this final move, therefore, I propose that care can be better understood as an indivisible part of "an ethics of worlding" (Barad, 2007, p. 392), or as I prefer to think of it, as part of a dynamic, entangled process of *responding to a world becoming.*

RESPONDING TO A WORLD-BECOMING OR POSTHUMANIZING RESPONSIVE EVALUATION

How does posthumanism help me rethink my ongoing concern for designing interactions that are inclusive and respectful of difference? Must I reject my commitments to understanding as a dialogical achievement, and the process through which we "grasp the character of our ethical responsibility" (George, 2014, p. 103)? At this stage in my posthumanist shift, although hesitant, my answer is no; rejection is not required, but a further decentering of the human is.

Drawing from philosopher Theodore George's (2014) presentation of Gadamer's philosophical project as one that calls for humans "to 'elevate' ourselves 'to humanity' through 'the aptitude... for conversation'" (p. 103), I will show how the intention behind such a call can support the agential materialism of posthumanism. George explains that the hermeneutic emphases evident in Heidegger and Gadamer's different, yet overlapping, theories, have always prioritized the possibilities inherent in our being beings-in-the-world, and as such "we remain answerable to being itself as it confronts us in the exteriority of our involvement with beings in always contingent, and, therefore, ever incalculable, shifting, and inimitably unique circumstances" (George, p. 107).

But how are we to enact this potentiality of being to be both "answerable to being" and become something other than what we perceive ourselves to be? George explains that for Heidegger "the scope and limits of human possibility are not determined by a presumed and pre-given essence... [but arise] ever anew in our involvement with beings encountered in the always singular and dynamic situations into which we are thrown" (p. 107). In other words, one could read this encounter as the posthuman entangled field from which the differentiating process of becoming human is enacted. Although Gadamer has been criticized for embracing the humanism Heidegger rejected, his rehabilitation of the humanist ideals of human responsibility and renewal enabled him to further develop Heidegger's critique of modernism. In doing so, he demonstrates that it is this capacity "to go beyond our particularity, to take into account the heritage... [and] grow above our limited selves" (Grondin, 1997, p. 164) that lends support to a posthumanist conception of humanism. This is because, for Gadamer, every dialogical encounter presents a challenge, as well as an opportunity, for us to rethink and reimagine our understandings of ethical life. It is in dialogue with others, in person, and across time and place, where what we are, can be, and can become are enacted, transformed, challenged, and renewed (George, 2014; Grondin, 1997). As such, it is in, and through, dialogue that we—humanity and world—become together. Philosopher Andrzej Wierciński (2011) illustrates:

> A conversation with the other does not primarily lead neither to an agreement, especially in regard to what is universal in our human experience of the world we live in nor to a nourishing of our individuality, but toward a community which we can patiently build and share in spite of our specific understandings and misunderstandings. (p. 55)

It is precisely because we have this capacity to participate in our own creation and recreation that humans have been, and always will be, considered agents. But I have come to believe that we do damage to ourselves and to the world around us when we consider agency as something only humans have to act with, and when our actions stand outside and above a world, a practice, or another being as something or someone we can choose to converse with or choose to ignore. I hold onto Gadamer's dialogical approach because he understood that our engagement in what matters already presupposes a need to be attentive to the subject matter or issue that pushes us from ourselves and towards that which is demanding our attention. Furthermore, he understood that the ethical demands of each encounter must always be addressed from within the encounter itself, and that for this encounter to be successful, it requires a giving oneself over to the movement of understanding itself and a willingness to be transformed in the process (Davey, 2013).

However, in the practice of responsive evaluation, the nature of the issues and the range of real and potential areas of disagreement make dialoguing across difference quite difficult to achieve. Even though it is understood that critical dialogue involves risk, a human-centered approach puts too much emphasis on what each individual means, intends, believes, has articulated or not articulated, has experienced or not experienced, and so on, and not enough on what is being materialized in the encounters. The focus on human agency, regardless of our assumptions about each other, always places some presumed notion of sameness or difference as abling or disabling responsive interaction, or as a marker of whether or not we can understand each other. While positive and productive dialogue among stakeholders does occur and will always be part of what we do, human-centered approaches tend to place more emphasis on the nature and quality of the relationships built between the people involved and on the nature and quality of what each individual brings to the table rather than on the development of the issue itself. It seems worth considering, therefore, an approach that moves beyond human responsiveness to one where all perspectives, human and nonhuman alike, are viewed as worthy partners in eliciting the matters that matter to the issue at hand.

A posthumanist turn does not deny our agency, or our capacity to "listen to the other," it simply does not presume that agency is located *in* any entity, whether human or nonhuman. Agency, and its role in materializing that which is considered meaningful, is an effect of the discursive practices that participate in forming and performing what we take to be important components of the world. In Barad's (2007) words:

> Discursive practices are not speech acts. Rather, discursive practices are specific material configurings of the world through which determinations of boundaries, properties, and meanings are differentially enacted... In my posthumanist account, meaning is not a human-based notion; rather, meaning is an ongoing performance of the world in its differential intelligibility. (p. 335)

Barad's agential materialism does not seek to eliminate differences. Rather her agential realist approach seeks to help us differentiate between differences that matter from those that matter less, or don't matter at all. As evaluators we are in the business of judging the value or worth of things which often requires a nuanced assessment of evidence as being "good" or "bad," "better," or "worse," "appropriate," or "inappropriate," in other words, variations of performances that matter. An agential realist approach takes the concern for relational practice mentioned earlier and turns it into something we as participants in the entangled becoming of the world must make sense of. Since matter is always, already entangled, an agential realist approach helps us make visible how "boundaries, properties, and meanings are differentially enacted through the intra-activity of mattering" (Barad, 2007, p. 392). In such an approach, Barad (2012) explains: "'responsibility' is not about right response, but rather a matter of inviting, welcoming, and enabling the response of the Other. That is, what is at issue is response-ability—the ability to respond" (p. 81).

Enabling Response-Ability in Encounters With Others

Merel Visse, Tineke Abma, and Guy Widdershoven (2015) ask: "What exactly does a responsive evaluator do and live by when he or she is *responsive to practices of responsibility*?" (p. 14, emphasis in original). I wish I had a simple answer. Gadamer has helped us understand that our capacity for continuous transformation through dialogical encounters requires that we "respond properly to the impetuses to understand that confront us in the course of our involvements" (George, 2014, p. 110). Care, reconceptualized as an ontological, political, and reflective practice (Hamington, 2014; Tronto, 1993), orients us to thinking of it as a fundamental part of evaluating ourselves as agents of obligation towards one another, rather than looking outside ourselves for principles or rules of conduct to follow. From these perspectives, we have come to understand that who we are is directly implicated with how we act and interact with others. It follows, then, that intervening in our practices of engagement and responsibility deserves reconsideration from a posthumanist stance.

The configurations that become stabilized in our institutions and programs are political. Not only do they actively participate in the defining and dispersion of care, they also purposefully or unwittingly serve to reproduce and create unfounded assumptions about certain people in ways that seep into our histories and resurface in our interactions and practices of engagement. The opening vignette is a good example of the way such assumptions get appropriated and recirculated as meaningful. Dialogue when conceived as a linguistic manifestation of our values, prejudices, and traditions becomes a participant in our practices of engagement. When dialogue is assumed to mediate between the world and our human understandings, it separates us from the world of which we are a part. Posthumanism provides a way to conceptualize dialogue as a participant in materializing what matters in the ongoing intra-actions between materializing entities. Different intra-actions will bring about the materialization and dematerialization of different phenomenal entities—for example, in the opening vignette, different levels of responsiveness to others, variations of care (e.g., protective, democratic (Tronto, 2016)), interpretations of meanings, bodily interactions, and so on, come and go as they intra-act with other matter. There is no definite, predetermined ethical stance to be taken in this approach, only possibility and potentialities for new connections, and new commitments (Barad, 2011).

Barad (2007) suggests a diffractive methodology "to study the entangled effects differences make" (p. 73). If we think about this analytically, our usual practice is to gather information and to examine that information in relation to the evaluation or research questions guiding the project. A diffractive methodology asks us to work analytically from within an entanglement of meaning and matter. It works within and across multiple disciplines as a way to better understand the way different discursive and material fields participate in boundary-making, relation-building, and other forms of worlding. Furthermore, it reveals how different methodological approaches participate in bringing-into-being different realities, and therefore different networks of effects. In such a way, it also helps us understand that dialogue is itself a participant in producing a certain kind of reality; a participant in the form meaning takes. As such, it must also be re-examined for what and how it produces, and who and what gets entangled in its actualization, and, in turn, how it might be actualized differently.

If responsibility involves having the potential to respond to a world-becoming, how do we enact this potential in evaluation design? What might a redesigning of the moral landscape of the first encounter at the museum look like? If taking a posthumanist stance means we assume that all entities, whether human or nonhuman, have inherent capacities to act and interact, what is our responsibility as human partners to materializing what matters in such encounters? How can our nonhuman partners make themselves known, and how do we account for their presence? Barad (2007) explains: "Responsibility is not ours alone. And yet our responsibility is greater than it would be if it were ours alone. Responsibility entails an ongoing responsiveness to the entanglements of self and other, here and there, now and then" (p. 394). It is, therefore, an event that requires participation. And participation, in whatever form it takes, still requires, it seems, that participants recognize its value and acknowledge that all entities intra-acting at any moment are active participants in the generative process put forward.

THE MUSEUM ENCOUNTER RE-IMAGINED

This was our first meeting with the Young Docents' Club (YDC), a museum-based, academic program for African-American teens in the Northeast. There were nine teens: four boys at one end of the long table and five girls at the other. Gail, the educational coordinator and former YDC coordinator was there, as well as Cynda, the brand new YDC coordinator. I was there, along with classmates from a course on participatory evaluation, to learn to conduct an evaluation by doing one. Since there were six of us forming the evaluation team, we scattered ourselves around the table so as not to form an obvious "them and us" division. Cynda suggested we all introduce ourselves, which we did. We then passed out large sheets of paper, sticky notes and index cards, as well as markers and pens. We explained to everyone that we had volunteered our services to the museum as a way to gain experience and learn about evaluation as a practice, and thanked them for letting us introduce the project. We stated that we believed that part of the process had to involve a way of generating ideas and questions about what it was we were evaluating, and how we might go about conducting the evaluation. Because we don't know them or the nature of their relationships, and they don't know us or the nature of our relationships, and because we do not know what might matter to each one of them, we felt that one way to begin was to work from where we were—and make the best of the formality of our meeting and the circumstance that brought us together. We invited them to jot down questions they might have about us, or to think about their experience thus far at the museum, to consider what they think an outsider might want to know about that experience or about the museum as a particular kind of place. We invited them to write, list, sketch or draw some aspect of that experience, and we did the same.

I was not surprised when some dove right into the activity while others sat back and watched. As we wrote or drew, I took note of the location of the meeting, the way the conference table created a wide distance between us. I wondered about the teens' lives outside these walls. Whether the museum had always been a familiar go-to place or was itself a new kind of experience. I began to draw the event we found ourselves in, exaggerating the scale of the institutional furniture and reducing the people to question marks. On the walls of my drawn room I wrote several questions: "What is a museum?," "What social and cultural artifacts are brought together in its space?," "Why do we care about how it might show up in the teens' lives?," and "How might we learn about what matters to them, and to the museum staff?" I noticed others participating as well. One girl became very involved with her drawing seemingly of herself in a museum gallery with children laughing all around her, while a boy was generating a list of things that mattered—"the mineral display," "I get paid for learning," "the friends I am making." Gail took the activity as an opportunity to write a list of all the things she was going to miss about working with the teens, and Cynda kept twirling her pen in the air with a look of consternation as if too many ideas were bombarding her at once.

As people drew and wrote, some of us gathered the finished products and began taping them around the room. We then invited everyone to read and use sticky notes to generate new questions and concerns. Although it was a tight fit and some of us were noticeably sweating even though the January wind could be felt through the single window, people were engaging. As people read, wrote, and talked about what they were seeing, I could feel new partners enter the scene—"fun," "appreciation," "care," "interest." And then "relationships" as some of the teens began to work together to add a note or story, or began to tease or poke at each other. Although they responded readily to Gail's glance, I took note of other partners—"expectations," "appropriate conduct," "care," "leadership." I also began taking notes of points of overlap, moments of confusion or tension, places where ideas and questions seemed to clash, all of which could potentially become points of entry for future engagement, questions, and invitations to generate more data or to analyze what we had. As the process generated a mixture of responses—drawings, stories, concerns, ideas, questions—we took pictures of the display telling them that we would like to continue the process next time. As the teens left for the day along with Gail and Cynda, I felt energized by the process and interested in hearing what my teammates were feeling and thinking. As some of my teammates began to collect the pile of notes and drawings we had generated, we were pleasantly surprised when Cynda poked her head back in the room and mentioned that the teens had invited us to observe their activities in the museum galleries the next week.

KEY CONCEPTS

- posthumanism
- dialogue
- difference
- responsive enactments
- world becoming

DISCUSSION QUESTIONS

1. The author amends Joan Tronto's (2013) statement that care, as a human expression, "always expresses an action or a disposition, a reaching out to something" (Tronto, 2013, p. x). Instead, she proposes to see care as intra-active (Barad, 2007): carer, cared-about, being cared for all "come to matter, in the very terms of the encounter" (Johns-Putra, 2013, p. 129). How do you perceive this yourself? What would this mean for your scholarly work?
2. What might a posthumanist turn in evaluation mean for how we conceptualize "validity" in evaluation?
3. How would you answer the question on what a responsive evaluator does and lives by "when he or she is responsive to practices of responsibility" (Visse, Abma, Widdershoven, 2015, p. 14)?

NOTE

1. All names for the program and individuals involved are pseudonyms

REFERENCES

Barad, K. (2003). Posthumanist performativity: Toward an understanding of how matter comes to matter. *Signs: Journal of Women in Culture and Society, 28*(3), 801–831.

Barad, K. (2007). *Meeting the universe halfway: Quantum physics and the entanglement of matter and meaning.* Durham, NC: Duke University Press.

Barad, K. (2011). Nature's queer performativity. *Qui Parle: Critical Humanities and Social Sciences, 19*(2), 121–158.

Barad K. (2012). Intra-actions [Interview with Adam Kleinman]. *Mousse Magazine, 34,* 76–81.

Burbules, N., & Rice, S. (1991). Dialogue across differences: Continuing the conversation. *Harvard Educational Review, 61*(4), 393–417.

Carr, W., & Kemmis, S. (1986). *Becoming critical: Education, knowledge and action research.* Philadelphia, PA: The Falmer Press.

Davey, N. (2013). *Unfinished worlds: Hermeneutics, aesthetics and Gadamer.* Edinburgh, Scotland: Edinburgh University Press.

Delpit, L. D. (1988). The silenced dialogue: Power and pedagogy in educating other people's children. *Harvard Educational Review, 58*(3), 280–298.

Eze, E. C. (2001). *Achieving our humanity: The idea of a postracial future.* New York, NY: Routledge.

Fry, T. (2011). *Design as politics.* New York, NY: Berg.

Gadamer, H.-G. (1989). *Truth and method* (2nd revised ed., J. Weinsheimer & D. G. Marshall, Trans.). New York, NY: Continuum.

Gadamer, H.-G. (2000). Subjectivity and intersubjectivity, subject and person. *Continental Philosophy Review, 33*(3), 275–287.

George, T. (2014). The responsibility to understand. In G.-J. van der Heiden (Ed.), *Phenomenological perspectives on plurality* (pp. 103–120). Leiden, Netherlands: Brill.

Gilpin, L. S. (2006). Postpositivist realist theory: Identity and representation revisited. *Multicultural Perspectives, 8*(4), 10–16.

Grondin, J. (1997). Gadamer on humanism. In L. E. Hahn (Ed.), *The philosophy of Hans-Georg Gadamer* (pp. 157–170). Peru, IL: Open Court Publishing Company.

Hamington, M. (2014). Care as Personal, Political, and Performative. In G. Olthuis, H. Kohlen, & J. Heier (Eds.), *Moral boundaries redrawn: The significance of Joan Tronto's argument for professional ethics, political theory and care practice* (pp. 195–212). Leuven, Belgium: Peeters in Leuven.

Johns-Putra, A. (2013). Environmental care ethics: Notes toward a new materialist critique. *Symploke, 21*(1–2), 125–135.

Kohn, M. (2000). Language, power, and persuasion: Toward a critique of deliberative democracy. *Constellations, 7*(3), 408–429.

Kushner, S. (2000). *Personalizing evaluation.* Thousand Oaks, CA: SAGE.

Lather, P. (1991). *Getting smart: feminist research and pedagogy with/in the postmodern.* New York, NY: Routledge.

Levinas, E. (1991). *Totality and infinity: An essay on exteriority.* Norwell, MA: Kluwer Academic.

Richardson, F. C. (2003). Virtue ethics, dialogue, and "reverence." *American Behavioral Scientist, 47*(4), 442–458.

Schmidt, D. J. (2012). On the sources of ethical life. *Research in Phenomenology, 42,* 35–48.

Schmidt, L. K. (2000). Respecting others: The hermeneutic virtue. *Continental Philosophy Review, 33,* 359–379.

Smith, M. K. (1994). *Local education: Community, conversation, praxis.* Buckingham, England: Open University Press.

Stake, R. E. (1975). To evaluate an arts program. In R. E. Stake (Ed.), *Evaluating the arts in education: A responsive approach* (pp. 13–31). Columbus, OH: Merrill.

Todd, S. (2009). Can there be pluralism without conflict? *Philosophy of Education Yearbook,* 51–59.

Tronto, J. (1993). *Moral boundaries: A political argument for an ethic of care.* New York, NY: Routledge.

Tronto, J. C. (2013). *Caring democracy: Markets, equality, and justice.* New York, NY: New York University Press.

Tronto, J. C. (2016). Protective care or democratic care? Some reflections on terrorism and care. [Comments prepared for presentation at SIGNAL, Cifas].

Visse, M., Abma, T., & Widdershoven, G. (2015). Practising political care ethics: Can responsive evaluation foster democratic care? *Ethics and Social Welfare, 9*(2), 164–182. doi:10.1080/17496535.2015.1005550

Wadsworth, Y. (2001). Becoming responsive—and some consequences for evaluation as dialogue across difference. *New Directions for Evaluation, 92,* 45–58.

Wierciński, A. (2011). "Sprache ist Gespräch": Gadamer's understanding of language as conversation. In A. Wierciński (Ed.), *Gadamer's hermeneutics and the art of conversation* (pp. 37–58). Münster, Germany: LIT Verlag.

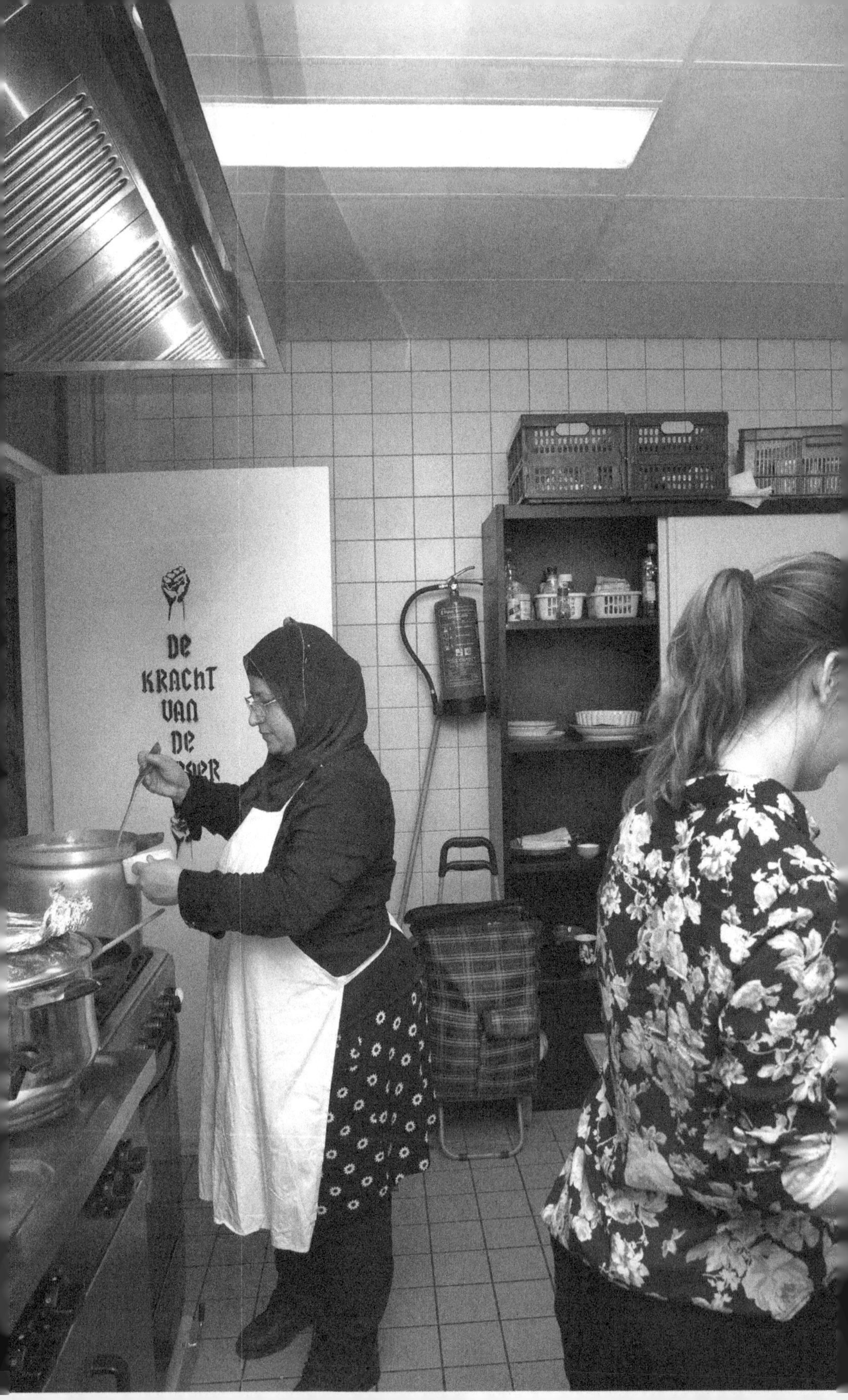

DE
KRACHT
VAN
DE

CHAPTER 9

RESPONSIVE EVALUATION AS A WAY TO CREATE SPACE FOR SEXUAL DIVERSITY

A Case Example on Gay-Friendly Elderly Care

Hannah Leyerzapf, Merel Visse,
Arwin de Beer, and Tineke Abma
VU Medical Center

In the Netherlands, three residential elderly care homes in two major cities collaborated in a responsive evaluation on gay-friendly elderly-care. Worldwide, being homosexual was long considered a religious sin and a psychological and medical abnormality, as well as illegal (Bitterman & Hess, 2016; Keuzenkamp, 2011). From around the turn of the twenty-first century onwards it seems that, at least in Europe and North America, lesbian, gay, bisexual, and transgender (LGBT)[1] people are gaining entrance to mainstream society and social acceptance is increasing (Bitterman & Hess, 2016). In a care context, as more and more people attain old age and an

Evaluation for a Caring Society, pages 207–223

increasing number of LGBT people are open about their sexual identity a 'new' population demographic of older LGBT people is established (Bitterman & Hess, 2016). Addis, Davies, Greene, MacBride-Stewart, & Shepherd (2009) report, however, that the understanding of older LGBT people's needs with regard to their health, social care, and housing is low and that research on this is scarce.

Internationally, the Netherlands has a reputation as a place of sexual freedom and emancipation (Hekma & Duyvendak, 2011), and equal rights for Dutch LGBT people are ensured by law. In practice, however, equity of people according to sexual orientation appears ambiguous as discrimination of LGBT people in society is reported to be increasing (Keuzenkamp, 2011; Keuzenkamp, Kooiman, & Van Lisdonk, 2012; Kuyper, 2015). In relation to health care, studies show that older LGBT people in the Netherlands postpone entering residential care as long as possible for fear of stigmatization and marginalization (Keuzenkamp, 2011; Schuyf, 1996, 2006, 2011). Estimates are that around 10% of the residents of elderly care homes are LGBT (Movisie, 2017). However, when asked about LGBT residents, management and care professionals of care homes stated not to "have" them or not to have "any problems with homosexuality," and increasing discrimination and exclusion turned out to be an unknown subject to them which they had not thought of before. This seems to fit the popular belief in Dutch society that tolerance for sexual diversity is widely spread, as well as a general public and political idea that equality of all Dutch people is reality and renders specific attention and sensitivity towards minority groups in society unnecessary (Essed & Hoving, 2014; Hekma, 1998; Hekma & Duyvendak, 2011).

Social interaction, participation, and empowerment of older people in the local context of the care home are of central importance to their wellbeing and quality of life (Barnes, 2005; Wahl & Weisman, 2003). Responsive evaluation can contribute to this as it is situated, aims to integrate multiple stakeholder perspectives, and hence is embedded. Several studies make a plea for empirical research involving elderly care organizations and the residents, care staff, and management to seek ways to address and deal with sexual diversity in daily practice and study how to increase participation and inclusion of older LGBT people in these contexts (Brotman, Ryan, & Cormier, 2003; Johnson, Jackson, Arnette, & Koffman, 2005; Simpson et al., 2015). In our responsive evaluation we therefore focused on gay-friendly care in three residential elderly care homes with the aim to shed light on the seeming, striking discrepancies between formal and theoretical/ideological space for sexual diversity and the informal, actual space in practice. This chapter first describes the approach and method of our evaluation and continues with a discussion of the main findings. Subsequently we will highlight topics that evaluators need to take into consideration when it concerns inclusion of sexual diversity in elderly care, looked at from a critical intersectionality and critical care ethical perspective (Bozalek, 2011; Zembylas, Bozalek, & Shefer, 2014; Hankivsky, 2014).

RESPONSIVE EVALUATION OF GAY-FRIENDLY ELDERLY CARE

All three homes that participated in our evaluation have been awarded with the Pink Passkey Award for gay-friendly care.[2] In 2008, an initiative was started by the nation-wide advocacy network for LGBT older people to create awareness in care homes and to stimulate action, which is then positively certified by an award. The so-called *Pink Passkey Award* can be acquired by care homes when they are gay-friendly in several areas, including activities for LGBT older adults, training for professionals, and focus on sexual diversity within policy and human resource management. One home that participated in our evaluation was the first to receive this award in 2008 and, together with one of the other two homes, is seen as a good example of sexual diversity management by national advocates. The third home acquired the award more recently (2015). These settings have been selected according to critical case sampling (Onwuegbuzie & Leech, 2007), as we aimed to select cases of care homes that would produce critical insight and learning potential on sexual diversity policies and practices.

The evaluation pays special attention to the involvement of multiple stakeholders in the evaluation process (Abma & Widdershoven, 2005; Abma, 2006; Greene, 2001). It has an inclusive agenda and aims to facilitate a mutual understanding on care practices from the perspectives of different stakeholder groups, particularly involving those who are structurally less heard and have less voice than those in more acknowledged power positions in the research setting (Abma, 2005; Baur, Abma, & Widdershoven, 2005). Through valuing of and reporting on the lived experiences of stakeholders, responsive evaluation aims to create conditions for multiple stakeholders' active contribution to practice development. In this study preliminary insights were shared with stakeholders in order for them to immediately translate findings into practice. Also, we carried out this evaluation by a cyclical process of data collection and analysis in which findings of earlier phases are input and guidance for subsequent phases (Denzin & Lincoln, 2005).

We collaborated in a team of three professional evaluators and an evaluation partner who is an experiential expert in the field of LGBT (i.e., is involved in advocacy groups and education activities on LGBT rights and gay-straight-alliances, and who identifies as LGBT). The professional evaluators carried out the data collection and analysis (Leyerzapf, Visse, De Beer,

& Abma, 2016). The evaluation partner critically followed these steps and provided feedback on analysis and reports and joined the meetings of the evaluators. The value of involving research or evaluation partners in scientific research and evaluation has been increasingly acknowledged (Abma, Nierse, & Widdershoven, 2009; Schipper, 2012; Schipper et al., 2010). Experiential knowledge complements the academic perspective and contributes to the quality of evaluation in various ways as evaluators engage with contextual values and norms (Abma & Broerse, 2010; Caron-Flinterman, Broerse, & Bunders, 2005). It helped to ground our evaluation in the experiences of participants and it also improved data interpretation and dissemination. An advisory group consisting of 11 representatives of organizations for older people in residential care and LGBT older adults in particular monitored the study and was asked for input and feedback throughout the study. The members were selected for their position in the field of LGBT elderly care. The advisory group contributed to the quality of the study and the development of recommendations for practice.

We included older LGBT people and older heterosexual people, as well as both LGBT and heterosexual care professionals, management and members of the client council of the care homes. An amount of 16 semi-structured, in-depth interviews, approximately 100 hours of participant observations of diverse activities within the care homes, and five focus groups were carried out. The participant observations, performed by the conducting researcher, focused on gaining insight on the content and form of activities for older LGBT as well as heterosexual people, the atmosphere, styles of communication, and social interactions. We attended chat groups and discussion groups, afternoons with music and sing-a-longs, movie nights, reminiscence groups, and educational theatre. Due to the invisibility of older LGBT adults and the sensitivity of our subject, these participant observations proved an important part of the evaluation as it enabled informal conversations with the participants, establishing trust and getting a sense of social norms enacted.

Focus groups (46 participants across five groups) were organized to validate and deepen our findings. The groups lasted between 1 and 2 hours, were held in the care homes, and chaired by a member of the research team or a professional of the care home in the presence of one of the researchers. Some focus groups included only older LGBT participants, others, called dialogue groups (Abma, 2001, 2003), included in some cases LGBT and heterosexual participants, and in other cases both heterosexual and LGBT residents and professionals (Krueger & Casey, 2000). These dialogue groups were relevant to reflect on gathered insights from a multistakeholder perspective and to develop mutual understanding (Berg & Lune, 2004; Bernard, 2011). The focus groups were organized according to a protocol designed by the evaluation team on the basis of the topic list used in the interviews and on insight gained from interviews and observations. Thematic outcomes of the interviews and observations were introduced to open the joint reflection. For a detailed report on the findings of the evaluation, including data analysis and quality criteria, we refer you to another publication (Leyerzapf et al., 2016).

DISCUSSION OF MAIN FINDINGS: FOUR THEMES

Lacking Awareness: Putting Sexual Diversity on the Agenda

Most heterosexual participants, as well as some LGBT professionals, were unfamiliar with the isolated and marginalized position of LGBT older people in care. Some referred to the dominant public image in the Netherlands being tolerant and progressive on individual freedom and sexual diversity, as a manager who said: "It shocked me actually. I didn't know about it... that [LGBT] elderly in care homes were in such a bad situation. I thought this couldn't happen in the Netherlands."[3] An LGBT staff member said: "People believe we don't need it, [they say:] 'we're done'—because we have gay marriage and the Gay Pride!" A heterosexual staff member stressed heterosexual people's unfamiliarity—in fact, pointing out their "otherness"—with LGBT (older) people in general: "For many, LGBT are men and women from Mars!" Older LGBT participants, some of which residents, and some care professionals told that awareness-raising on the position of LGBT older people should be first priority in care homes. With this objective in mind, two of the care homes initiated specific training for care professionals, and all three homes organized activities for heterosexual and LGBT residents, visitors and care professionals to bring the topic to the attention. The professionals advocating sexual diversity stressed the necessity of its structural integration in the care homes as including structural focus in organization vision and policy and installing central contact people. The questions is, however, if such a focus on structure is enough to generate change for LGBT (older) people.

Social Exclusion, (In)visibility and Difference

For LGBT participants daily reality was characterized by experiences of stigmatization and social exclusion by heterosexual residents or staff of the care home, out of fear for which they reported to feel forced to keep their sexual orientation a secret. An older LGBT male recounted: "For example, they [other residents] wouldn't sit next to me at dinner or coffee." An

LGBT female resident reported that she was often met with name-calling by older people in her care home: "They call me a dyke." Other LGBT participants told of stigmatizing humor, such as older heterosexual people or staff telling jokes equating homosexuality with promiscuous behavior because of an overly sexually explicit appearance as LGBT men dressed in tight black leather pants or wearing a thong at the Gay Canal Pride. LGBT participants recounted of peers or themselves to have had recurrent experiences with being discriminated against for their supposed sexual orientation throughout their lives. They have had to learn to hide their sexual orientation at work or even from their families and social circle. Some tried to mold themselves and their sexuality in such a way that they fit normal (i.e., heterosexual) lifestyles and identities. Some argued their sexual orientation is not interesting because it's "just" a private matter. In both cases participants seemed to want to be invisible (i.e., not stand out and not be different). Other LGBT participants, however, said they deliberately chose to be open about their sexual orientation because they refuse to obscure their true identity. They seemed to present themselves in a deliberate activist style and often had been involved in activist movements as they were younger. They seemed to be (hyper)visible as (older) LGBT and consciously celebrating this difference. The hidden or overly visible lives of the LGBT participants pointed to a status quo culture in which heterosexuality and specific identities and lifestyles in which these are supposedly reflected is the norm, and everything deviating from that is different, thus not normal.

Safety, Feeling at Home and Being (Accepted as) Yourself

All LGBT participants expressed the need to feel safe, accepted, and at home as well as to be able to "be themselves" in their care home. They explained this last point as both being able to do and choose what they consider valuable, and being socially acknowledged and respected in this. Many felt this is not possible while having to stay secretive about their sexual orientation. They stated that the LGBT activities really make a difference as they provide a safe space to meet like-minded people and share and exchange personal experiences and emotions. Staff involved in LGBT activities told that some participants speak in these activities about their sexual orientation, their life story, and painful memories of exclusion *for the first time in their life.* LGBT participants spoke of a sense of individual and collective strength they feel when sharing their experiences with others who have similar life stories, and described feelings of collective belonging and being at home—captured in that some called the people in these discussion groups their extended family. An older LGBT man, regular visitor of the weekly Pink Salon in one of the care homes, explained: "In the last few years... I really have become more outspoken. I have become the person I really am now... [someone] that speaks up. This is connected with the way people communicate there; everything is said out in the open. It was a sort of coming home as well. I can... be myself there."

LGBT participants, as well as involved care professionals, stated that for the LGBT activities to support LGBT to feel safe, home-like and empowered a respectful, inclusive atmosphere and manner of communication are essential, as well as development of mutual trust (i.e., between heterosexual and LGBT in the care home). LGBT staff stressed that they felt that to ensure participation and inclusion of LGBT older people in the homes "for the long run," actions and policy need to go beyond exclusive, categorical activities and address the structural organization and culture of the home. At the same time, however, older LGBT and LGBT and heterosexual staff, emphasized that "homosexuality should not be made too explicit" as this would contribute to the visibility of the otherness of older LGBT people instead of adding to it being normal. In line with this, all LGBT participants repeatedly and urgently expressed that they are "foremost humans" and "we are people as well." In this the doubleness of striving for acknowledgement from an identity politics-inspired collective identity as well as for individual recognition as unique *and* equitable seems expressed, and participants seem to appeal to a balance between the two.

Corresponding Experiences and Needs of Older LGBT and Heterosexual People

Older *heterosexual* participants also reported that feeling safe and at home is essential in their daily life in the care home. To acquire this, both LGBT and heterosexual residents pointed out the importance of good interaction with and personal attention from staff. They said that it is often difficult to establish contact with fellow residents. Also, all participants made it clear that belonging and connectedness among residents is important in order to feel safe, at home, and well in the home. Staff and older heterosexual participants reported social segregation in the homes, and some of the latter experiences of hassling and name-calling as well. Also, LGBT *and* heterosexual participants experienced a taboo on intimacy and sexuality of older people, especially within the context of care relating to patients/clients. An older heterosexual resident non-understandingly said: "[Care professionals and care organizations] all believe love and intimacy among older people do not exist!" Nevertheless, some heterosexual participants seemed to support such a view when it came to LGBT older people by clearly expressing limits to visible expressions of love and intimacy other than "normal": "Of course you don't show it overtly."

Parallel experiences and needs of LGBT and heterosexual older people notwithstanding, professionals advocating LGBT inclusion in the three care homes worried about possibilities for change and future support for sexual diversity. Only in one of the homes was the professional assigned to advocate sexual diversity officially assigned as sexual diversity manager—the first and only one in the Netherlands. In the other homes two care professionals performed their work on an informal basis, i.e., acknowledged by the management but *secondary* to their primary activities. They themselves, as well as LGBT older people visiting the activities they organized, worried about the continuation of the attention for sexual diversity in the home should they leave.

PROMOTING SEXUAL DIVERSITY AS AN EVALUATOR: TOPICS TO CONSIDER

Enclave Deliberation—Othering

From our evaluation we learned that exclusive, sometimes explicitly announced, sometimes hidden, LGBT activities in care homes focusing on sharing experiences of exclusion, meet older LGBT people's needs to be with like-minded people and for safe, home-like spaces. This form of enclave deliberation (Karpowitz, Raphael, & Hammond, 2009) appears from participants' accounts on development of personal and relational empowerment (Rowlands, 1998), and supports and develops well-being and voice of LGBT people in these study settings. However, participants stated that they want to feel included, to belong and be personally acknowledged in the care home as a whole as well—signalling the need for connection with heterosexual residents and professionals as well as structural inclusion/participation in the organization. In part, enclave deliberation is needed because of the unsafe, exclusionary heteronormative and sometimes homophobic climate in the care homes and society in general. Bearing in mind processes of normalization of heterosexuality and the *othering* (Johnson et al., 2004) of everyone considered non-heterosexual, it is clear that structural and long-term empowerment and inclusion of LGBT people in residential care requires additional action and a move beyond a singular categorical approach to sexual diversity. Responsive evaluation can contribute crucially to this process by bringing together multi-stakeholder perspectives in critical dialogue. But how do we foster a process where dominant stakeholders make space for marginalized groups? For this, structural power relations (in)forming structure and culture in the care home or other evaluation setting, need to be taken into consideration.

Micro-Aggression, Normalization, and Non-Performativity

Within the Netherlands, where formal/legally-challengeable discrimination is rare, othering of LGBT people typically occur in an implicit, invisible, everyday way. The (c)overt discriminations or *micro-aggressions* experienced by LGBT participants, like name-calling and exclusionary humor, are difficult to pinpoint because heterosexual people are mostly unaware of the possible extensive, painful effects on LGBT people (Sue, 2010). This is due to the fact that they are deeply rooted in a dominant tradition of heteronormativity in society in which heterosexuality is normalized and institutionalized (Jackson, 2006). Therefore, micro-aggressions against LGBT people are difficult to resist and to address as the person that speaks up is often perceived as a nag or kill-joy (Ahmed, 2007; Essed, 1991; Sue, 2010). As normalization works both ways (Leyerzapf, Verdonk, Ghorashi, & Abma, 2017) older LGBT people are not only perceived as different by others/heterosexual people, but, to a certain extent, also perceive of themselves as such (Hekma & Duyvendak, 2011; Jackson, 2006). All this makes social exclusion in relation to sexual diversity, or diversity in general, a difficult issue to address and attention for and policy on sexual diversity often rhetorical and non-performative within organizations (Ahmed, 2015; Knoppers, Claringbould, & Dortants, 2015). Thus it is necessary that hidden or hypervisible experiences of differences are made visible first, and subsequently recognized and acknowledged as micro-aggressions, involving othering and constituting structural inequality (Leyerzapf et al., 2017).

Revealing Privilege/Disadvantage Through Critical Intersectionality

As heterosexuality signifies a privileged social status, it is crucial to address the selective privilege and disadvantage linked to heteronormativity. This constitutes the unearned advantage that—supposedly—heterosexual (older) people unawarely experience, enabling them to participate, belong, and exercise voice in the care home relatively easy as they are seen as/see themselves as representing or at least fitting the norm, while supposedly non-heterosexual (older) people or those openly identifying as LGBT experience disadvantage as they are seen as/see themselves as not representing or fitting the norm (i.e., as different/deviant). Willis, Maegusuku-Hewett, Raithby, &

Miles (2014) also point to the social power dynamics at play by describing care homes as "spaces in which heterosexual relationships, norms and milestones are routinely privileged over other sexual identities and desires" (p. 2).

The process of privileging occurs through normative discourses and social imaging, characterized by static, categorical, and stigmatized views on LGBT people, their sexuality, and specifically that of older LGBT people, and in which they become othered (Leyerzapf et al., 2017). Willis, Maegusuku-Hewett, Raithby, & Miles (2014) are reluctant to emphasize the needs of LGBT people as a separate category for fear of sustaining this categorical thinking. Indeed, in fact, identity aspects of sexual orientation, sexuality, gender, age, and ability all intersect and interact here in multiple and complex ways (Verdonk, Muntinga, Leyerzapf, & Abma, 2015). Although Hankivsky (2014) calls to overcome "naturalized essentialisms" in the context of diversity research or management, the route is not to avoid categorizations—as these entail an inherent human social function. Key is to unveil their hierarchical orderings and underlying systems of oppression and domination, and, involving the critical intersectionality lens, explore the "*synergistic* effects of [these] interlocking structures of power" (Hankivsky, 2014, p. 260, emphasis in original).

Challenging the normalization of privilege and disadvantage and the underlying social hierarchies, starts with practising critical reflexivity on one's own and dominant social norms. Reflexivity is a daily, ongoing process and dialectical act—not something that can be acquired and ticked off, but an awareness, sensitivity, and attitude that needs to be enacted and therefore is contextual and involves relating to "others." Parallel to this, critical dialogue is required in which multiple stakeholders meet and practice reflexivity in a structured way. For such a dialogue to actually come about, a temporary, safe space is required. This requires people to not only listen to each other but to commit themselves to the stories of the "others" and feel responsible—meaning a horizontal sharing of stories or *caring with* instead of a hierarchical, potentially paternalistic (caring) relationship (Zembylas, Bozalek, & Shefer, 2014). However, how can this be enacted within the context of existing privileged (ir)responsibility, affecting who cares or needs to care for and about whom and who does not (Zembylas, Bozalek, & Shefer, 2014)? Will people be prepared to give up privilege; the privilege of not having to care, to engage and to feel responsible, and give up space to "others"?

Balancing Equality and Equity, Sameness and Difference: Daring to Care via Narratives

The open, emergent as well as dialogical design of responsive evaluation supports the beyond-the-categorical-approach and helps to move away from a binary interpretation of power, and also for example, gender as oppositional, crucial for entering critical dialogue, and for developing reflexivity. In our evaluation it pointed out the parallels between experiences and needs of LGBT and heterosexual older people (in care), but it also brought forward the fact that some LGBT participants were reluctant to profile and be targeted in the care homes *as well as* within the evaluation as LGBT. They felt uncomfortable as they felt other identity aspects, that for some and/or in some contexts according to them were more relevant and meaningful, were left out and made them feel unacknowledged as a whole person. Aspects could be gender, class, partner status, religion, and so on. Caring "equally" and equity in care is not about equal treatment, participants told us (Willis et al., 2014). We learned, however, that being able to organize explicit *pink activities* (i.e., activities for LGBT people) in the care home and these being announced by hoisting of the rainbow flag on top of the home, answered the parallel wish of some for public, collective recognition and reclaiming of their equality and equal rights. Yet again, the appeal for equality via "difference" notwithstanding, many seemed to make an appeal for equity through sameness by emphasizing themselves as "being human" ("we are *foremost* humans").

The dialogical and biographical character of responsive evaluation can help to bring together and create space for these multiple, intersecting narratives. Also, it can facilitate coalition building and working towards strong, alliances across different differences (Hankivsky, 2014). This is important because diversity advocacy and policy action focused on different diversity aspects (gender, culture/ethnicity/race, sexual diversity) easily end up as an *oppression olympics*, and arrive at a deadlock of discussions about legitimacy of discrimination and oppression claims resulting in non-performativity (Ahmed, 2015; Hankivsky, 2014). Besides strategic essentialism tuned to situated context and collective objective(s) (Verdonk, Muntinga, Leyerzapf, & Abma, 2015), a balancing of sameness and difference is necessary in order to strike an effective balance between equality and equity and build recognition of a social collective, as well as as a personal, unique, and at the same time indivisible and fluid, person. With legal equality and consumer-hospitality in mind, Dutch residential care homes, as those in our evaluation, claim to be "open to everyone" and often deem it inappropriate to explicate sexual diversity and older LGBT people in their policy. This ideology that everybody is equal and should be treated the same is strong in the Netherlands but hinders positive, meaningful recognition of difference (Johnson et al., 2004; Ghorashi, 2010; Ghorashi & Sabelis, 2013). Being reflexive on (own) normativity includes recognizing existing practices in care homes as not neutral but reflecting dominant societal norms and hierarchies such as this *equality-as-sameness* discourse.

As stories are open for interpretation, critical dialogue on the basis of sharing of narratives enables to embrace differences and for people to practice alterity, that is, open up to the position of the other (Abma, 2003; Bozalek, 2011; Ghorashi & Sabelis, 2013). Then, if emotions and felt tensions, as resentment, guilt, shame, as well as accumulated pain and anger, are let in and openly discussed, contiguity and common ground can be experienced and mutuality, engagement, and shared responsibility developed (Abma 2001, 2003; Ghorashi & Sabelis, 2013). As we have seen in this evaluation, in dialogue between LGBT (older) people, heterosexual (older) people and professionals of care homes, personal stories of (anonymous) LGBT people could be presented to invoke reflections and reflexivity, and develop ideas about practice improvement. If in a safe climate heterosexual and LGBT older people could explore and find shared memories such as experiences of loneliness and loss due to aging. Involving narratives on intimacy and sexuality of older people could counter the *double invisibility* of LGBT older people (Simpson et al., 2015). Since feelings of agency and autonomy are closely interconnected with feelings of authenticity, a biographical approach, including both homogeneous and heterogeneous dialogue, in responsive evaluation can play a key role in empowerment and change (Cornelison & Doll, 2013; Willis et al., 2014). However, to start up the challenging, sensitive process of critical dialogue and practice of reflexivity, policy makers *and* responsive evaluators should set the example (Hankivsky, 2014). They are part of existing (hetero)normativity and need to confront their own privilege, the ways in which their norms are in- and ex-clusive and the social hierarchies on which these are based. In our evaluation this crystallized into the question posed to us as evaluators: Why are you, as heterosexual people, studying LGBT issues? More importantly, perhaps, evaluators and policy makers engaged in evaluation projects directed at inclusive, equitable care practices, should head in *daring to care* as they are moving from a mainstream position of relative voice and power and can engage in difficult, possibly uncomfortable reflections without risking actual emotional, social, material/physical consequences and giving up relative—limited, hidden—safe space as would LGBT (older) people have to do.

KEY CONCEPTS

- difference
- enclave deliberation
- micro agressions
- critical intersectionality
- critical care ethics

DISCUSSION QUESTIONS

1. What are the promises of critical intersectionality for evaluators?
2. The authors address the topic of *courage*, when they write "evaluators and policy makers . . . should head in *daring to care* as they are moving from a mainstream position of relative voice and power and can engage in difficult, possibly uncomfortable reflections." How can evaluators cultivate the courage to stay open and facilitate these kinds of difficult reflections?
3. The authors of this paper are based in the Netherlands. If you are not from the Netherlands, how do you experience the invisibility of LGBT people in residential elderly care homes? The participants of this study reported that they didn't want to stand out or be different. How can evaluators reach people to learn about what matters to them, when they'd rather not be seen?

NOTES

1. In international literature the terms *gay*, *LGBT(Q)(I)*, and *homosexual* are all used to designate older people who identify with a non-heterosexual and/or non-cisgender lifestyle and identity. Within the Netherlands, the terms *homosexuality* and *being homosexual* are most commonly used to address these identifications. In this chapter, for practicality, we use the term LGBT to signify all these possible identities, however, in the quotations of participants the terms homosexual and homosexuality are mostly left unchanged.
2. Parallel to the international development of gay-friendly care, in the Netherlands attention started to go out to "pink elderly care" (Hekma & Duyvendak, 2011; Keuzenkamp, 2011; Kuyper, Iedema, & Keuzenkamp, 2013). The color pink now positively signifies homosexuality in the Netherlands and is an identifying marker of many advocacy groups, however, it links back to LGBT adults being forced to wear a pink triangle during their collective persecution in World War II.
3. Sentences between double quotation marks are verbatim quotations of participants, translated from Dutch by the first author and checked by the second authors. Overall, as much as possible, words and expressions from participants were used to describe the findings.

REFERENCES

Abma, T. A. (2001). Reflexive dialogues: A story about the development of injury prevention in two performing art schools. *Evaluation, 7,* 238–252.

Abma, T. A. (2003). Learning by telling: Storytelling workshops as an organizational learning intervention. *Management Learning, 34,* 221–240.

Abma, T. A. (2005). Responsive evaluation: Its value and special contribution to health promotion. *Evaluation and Program Planning, 28,* 279–289.

Abma, T. A. (2006). The practice and politics of responsive evaluation. *The American Journal of Evaluation, 27,* 31–43.

Abma, T. A., & Broerse, J. E. W. (2010). Patient participation as dialogue: Setting research agendas. *Health Expectations, 13,* 160–73.

Abma, T. A., Nierse, C. J., & Widdershoven, G. A. (2009). Patients as partners in responsive research: Methodological notions for collaborations in mixed research teams. *Qualitative Health Research, 19,* 401–15.

Abma, T. A., & Widdershoven, G. A. M. (2005). Sharing stories: Narrative and dialogue in responsive nursing evaluation. *Evaluation and the Health Professions, 28,* 90–109.

Addis, S., Davies, M., Greene, G., MacBride-Stewart, S., & Shepherd, M. (2009). The health, social care and housing needs of lesbian, gay, bisexual and transgender older people: A review of the literature. *Health & social care in the community, 17,* 647–58.

Ahmed, S. (2007). The Language of Diversity. *Ethnic and Racial Studies, 30,* 235–256.

Ahmed, S. (2015, February 5). *Brick walls: Racism and other hard histories.* Difference that makes no Difference: The Non-Performativity of Intersectionality and Diversity. Oral communication at the International Workshop Frankfurt Research Center for Postcolonial Studies (FRCPS) in cooperation with the Womens' Network, Cluster of Excellence, Germany.

Barnes, M. (2005). The same old process? Older people, participation and deliberation. *Ageing & Society, 25,* 245–259.

Baur, V. E., Abma, T. A., & Widdershoven, G. A. M. (2010). Participation of marginalized people in evaluation: mission impossible? *Evaluation and Program Planning, 33,* 238–45.

Berg, B. L., & Lune, H. (2004). *Qualitative Research Methods for the Social Sciences.* Boston, MA: Pearson.

Bernard, H. R. (2011). *Research methods in anthropology: Qualitative and quantitative approaches.* Lanham, MD: Rowman AltaMira.

Bitterman, A., & Hess, D. B. (2016). Gay ghettoes growing gray: transformation of gay urban districts across north America reflects generational change. *The Journal of American Culture, 39,* 55–63.

Bozalek, V. (2011). Acknowledging privilege through encounters with difference: Participatory learning and action techniques for decolonising methodologies in Southern contexts. *International Journal of Social Research Methodology, 14,* 469–484. doi: 10.1080/13645579.2011.611383

Brotman, S., Ryan, B., & Cormier, R. (2003). The health and social service needs of gay and lesbian elders and their families in Canada. *The Gerontologist, 43,* 192–202.

Caron-Flinterman, J. F., Broerse, J. E. W., & Bunders, J. F. G. (2005). The experiential knowledge of patients: A new resource for biomedical research? *Social Science & Medicine, 60,* 2575–2584.

Cornelison, L. J., & Doll, G. M. (2013). Management of sexual expression in long-term care: Ombudsmen's perspectives. *The Gerontologist, 53,* 780–789.

Denzin, N. K., & Lincoln, Y. S. (Eds.). (2005). *The SAGE Handbook of Qualitative Research.* Thousand Oaks, CA: SAGE.

Essed, P. (1991). *Understanding everyday racism: An interdisciplinary theory.*Newbury Park, CA: SAGE.

Essed, P., & Hoving, I. (2014). Innocence, smug ignorance, resentment: An introduction to Dutch racism. In P. Essed, & I. Hoving. (Eds.), *Dutch racism* (pp. 9–30). Amsterdam, Netherlands: Rodopi.

Ghorashi, H. (2010). *Culturele Diversiteit, Nederlandse Identiteit en Democratisch Burgerschap* [Cultural diversity, Dutch identity and democratic citizenship]. Den Haag, Netherlands: Sdu.

Ghorashi, H., & Sabelis, I. (2013). Juggling difference and sameness: Rethinking strategies for diversity in organizations. *Scandinavian Journal of Management, 29,* 78–86.

Greene, J. C. (2001). Dialogue in evaluation a relational perspective. *Evaluation, 7,* 181–187.

Hankivsky, O. (2014). Rethinking care ethics: On the promise and potential of an intersectional analysis. *American Political Science Review, 108,* 252–264.

Hekma, G. (1998). As long as they don't make an issue of it… *Journal of Homosexuality, 35,* 1–23.

Hekma, G., & Duyvendak, J. W. (2011). Queer Netherlands: A puzzling example. *Sexualities, 14,* 625–31.

Jackson, S. (2006). Gender, sexuality and heterosexuality: The complexity (and limits) of heteronormativity. *Feminist Theory, 7,* 105–121.

Johnson, J. L., Bottorff, J. L., Browne, A. J., Grewal, S., Hilton, B. A., & Clarke, H. (2004). Othering and being othered in the context of health care services. *Health Communication, 16,* 255–71.

Johnson, M. J., Jackson, N. C., Arnette, J. K., & Koffman, S. D. (2005). Gay and lesbian perceptions of discrimination in retirement care facilities. *Journal of Homosexuality, 49,* 83–102.

Karpowitz, C. F., Raphael, C., & Hammond, A. S. (2009). Deliberative democracy and inequality: Two cheers for enclave deliberation among the disempowered. *Politics & Society, 37,* 576–615.

Keuzenkamp, S. (2011). *Acceptatie van Homoseksualiteit in Nederland 2011. Internationale Vergelijking, Ontwikkelingen en Actuele Situatie* [Acceptance of homosexuality in The Netherlands 2011. International comparison, developments and actual situation]. Den Haag, Netherlands: Sociaal en Cultureel Planbureau.

Keuzenkamp, S., Kooiman, N., & Van Lisdonk, J. (Eds.). (2012). *Niet te Ver uit de Kast. Ervaringen van Homo- en Biseksuelen in Nederland* [Not too far out of the closet: experiences of homosexual and bisexual people in The Netherlands]. Den Haag, Netherlands: Social en Cultureel Planbureau.

Knoppers, A., Claringbould, I., & Dortants, M. (2015). Discursive managerial practices of diversity and homogeneity. *Journal of Gender Studies, 24,* 259–74.

Krueger, R., & Casey, M. A. (2000). *Focus groups: A practical guide for applied research.* Thousand Oaks, CA: SAGE.

Kuyper, L. (2015). *Wel Trouwen, Niet Zoenen. De Houding van de Nederlandse Bevolking tegenover Lesbische, Homoseksuele, Biseksuele en Transgender Personen 2015* [Marry: yes, Kiss: no. The attitude of Dutch population toward homosexual, bisexual and transgender people in 2015]. Den Haag, Netherlands: Sociaal en Cultureel Planbureau.

Kuyper, L., Iedema, J., & Keuzenkamp, S. (2013). *Towards tolerance. Exploring changes and explaining differences in attitudes towards homosexuality in Europe.* Den Haag, Netherlands: Sociaal en Cultureel Planbureau.

Leyerzapf, H., Visse, M., De Beer, A., & Abma, T. A. (2016). Gay-friendly elderly care: Creating space for sexual diversity in residential care by challenging the hetero norm. *Ageing & Society*, 1–26. doi: 10.1017/S0144686X16001045.

Leyerzapf, H., Verdonk, P., Ghorashi, H., & Abma, T. (2017). *"We are all so different that it is just . . . normal." Normalization practices in an academic hospital in the Netherlands.* (Manuscript submitted for publication).

Movisie. (2017). *Ouderen en Homoseksualiteit* [The elderly and homosexuality]. Movisie, the Netherlands center for social development, Utrecht. Retrieved from www.movisie.nl.

Onwuegbuzie, A. J., & Leech, N. L. (2007). Sampling designs in qualitative research: Making the sampling process more public. *The Qualitative Report, 12,* 238–254.

Rowlands, J. (1998) A word of the times, but what does it mean? Empowerment in the discourse and practice of development. In H. Afshar (Ed.), *Women and empowerment: Illustrations from the Third World* (pp. 11–34). Basingstoke: Macmillan.

Schipper, K. (2012). *Patient participation and knowledge.* Amsterdam, Netherlands: VU University Press.

Schipper, K. T., Abma, A., Van Zadelhoff, E., Van de Griendt, J., Nierse, C., & Widdershoven, G. A. M. (2010). What does it mean to be a patient research partner? An ethnodrama. *Qualitative Inquiry, 16,* 501–510.

Schuyf, J. (1996). *Oud Roze. De Positie van Lesbische en Homoseksuele Ouderen in Nederland* [Old Pink: The position of lesbian and homosexual eldery in The Netherlands]. Utrecht, Netherlands: Publicatiereeks Homostudies Universiteit van Utrecht.

Schuyf, J. (2006). *Groenboek Belweek Roze Ouderen* [Greenbook CallWeek Pink Elderly]. Projectgroep Roze Ouderen: ANBO voor 50-plussers, COC Nederland, Schorer, Kenniscentrum Lesbisch- en Homo Emancipatiebeleid.

Schuyf, J. (2011). *Groenboek Belweek Roze Ouderen* [Greenbook CallWeek Pink Elderly]. Projectgroep Roze Ouderen: ANBO voor 50-plussers, COC Nederland, Schorer, Kenniscentrum Lesbisch- en Homo Emancipatiebeleid.

Simpson, P., Horne, M., Brown, L. J., Wilson, C. B., Dickinson, T., & Torkington, K. (2015). Old(er) care home residents and sexual/intimate citizenship. *Ageing and Society, 37,* 243–265. doi:10.1017/S0144686X15001105

Sue, D. W. (2010). *Microaggressions in everyday life: Race, gender, and sexual orientation.* Hoboken, NJ: John Wiley & Sons.

Verdonk, P., Muntinga, M., Leyerzapf, H., & Abma, T. (2015). Strategisch pendelen tussen gestolde categorieën en fluïde identiteiten. Dynamische verschillen in de zorg begrijpen en onderzoeken vanuit intersectionaliteitintersectionaliteit [Strategic balancing between fixed categories and fluid identities. Understanding and researching dynamic differences in care from intersectionality]. *Tijdschrift voor Genderstudies, 18,* 433–450.

Wahl, H. W., & Weisman, G. D. (2003). Environmental gerontology at the beginning of the new millenium: Reflections on its historical, empirical, and theoretical development. *The Gerontologist, 43,* 616–627.

Willis, P., Maegusuku-Hewett, T., Raithby, M., & Miles, P. (2016). Swimming upstream: The provision of inclusive care to older lesbian, gay and bisexual (LGB) adults in residential and nursing environments in Wales. *Ageing and Society, 36,* 282–306.

Zembylas, M., Bozalek, V., & Shefer, T. (2014). Tronto's notion of privileged irresponsibility and the reconceptualisation of care: implications for critical pedagogies of emotion in higher education. *Gender and Education, 26,* 200–214. doi: 10.1080/09540253.2014.901718

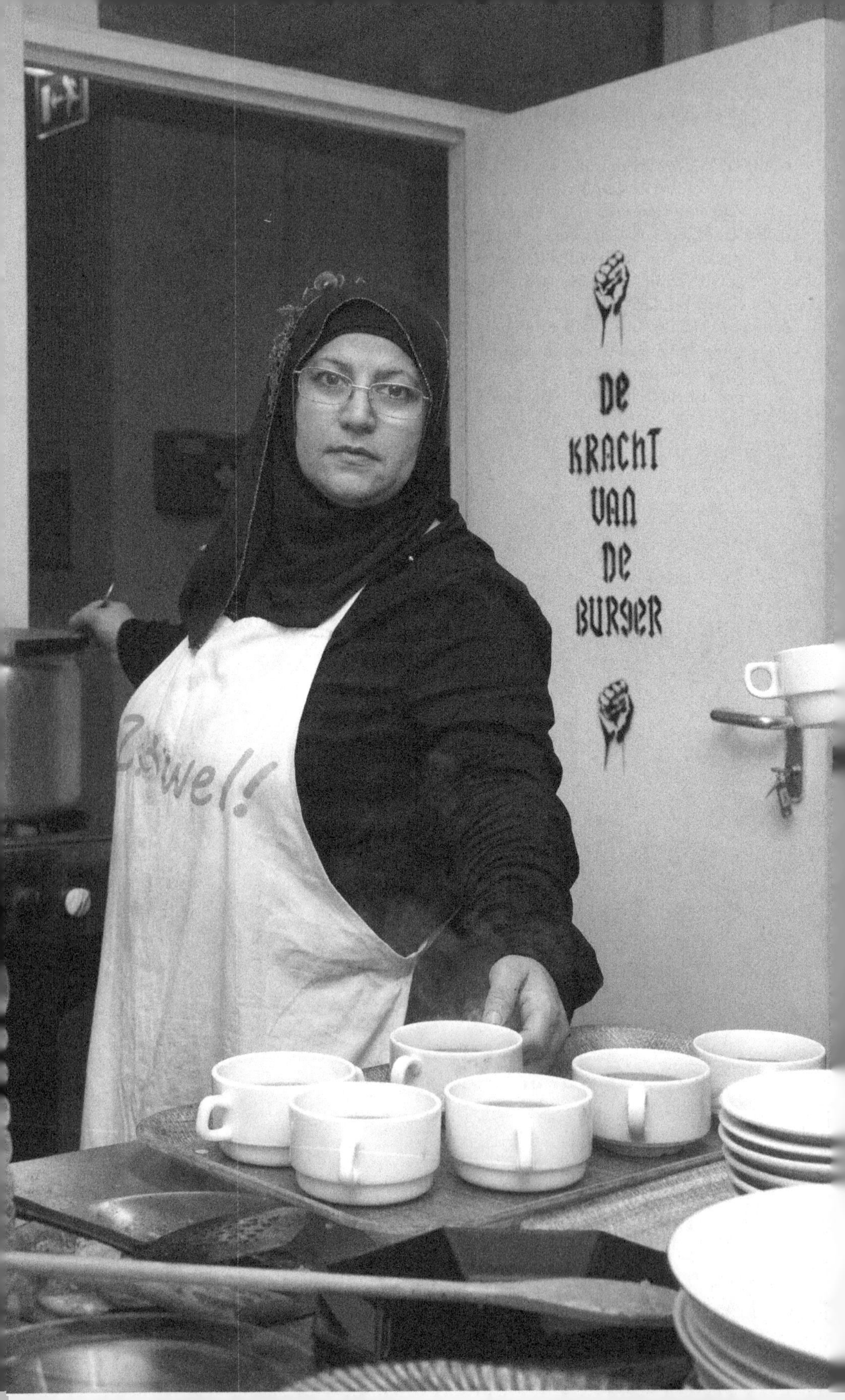
DE
KRACHT
VAN
DE
BURGER

CHAPTER 10

EVALUATION FOR A CARING SOCIETY

Toward New Imaginaries

Merel Visse and Tineke Abma
VU Medical Center

This volume highlights responsive, participatory, and democratic approaches to evaluation in the context of care. We aimed to learn how care can enrich evaluators' work to foster a caring society. Care regards society as the complex, relational engagement of people who do everything to maintain and repair their life-sustaining webs so that they can live their lives as well as possible (Fisher & Tronto, 1990, p. 40). While searching for more specific definitions, scholars in care ethics and care theory still discuss what care is: a skill or a virtue, a practice or a relational ontology. In our own work, we see care as a moral-political and creative practice of mutual learning that constitutes the ongoing unfolding and becoming of interdependent people who are part of nested relationships (Kittay, 1999; Leget, van Nistelrooij, & Visse, 2017; Visse, Abma, & Widdershoven, 2015).

Evaluation for a Caring Society, pages 225–242

This means that we do not see care primarily as a skill, virtue, or principle for which we should strive nor as solely as care work (e.g., cleaning, nursing, and cooking). Instead, we see care as a creative, relational approach to morality. Care emerges from what occurs in the particular, everyday situations of our society. Care has a liminal quality: It can exist in the spaces between people who collaborate in programs, policies, and practices, and it can be imagined, wished for when it is absent. In our view, evaluators ideally do not primarily focus on assessing or measuring the effectiveness of programs, policies, or practices by external standards. Instead, they relate to these practices from a care perspective. They humble their knowing through becoming part of these practices and seeing their work as a praxis of care itself.1 Only then can they become familiar with what matters to those dependent on the evaluated programs, policies, and practices and what their deepest concerns are. Evaluators thus leave the highlands and enter the complexities and messiness of practices, what Donald Schön (1991) calls the swampy lowlands.

In the following, we propose several foci for evaluators who work from a care perspective or wish to encourage a caring society. This is not a society that has a caring element, such as an activity, outcome, or evaluation (whether caring or not). Rather, this society sees care as a continuously unfolding relational praxis of moral-political learning that is central to the very fabric of society and is enacted through reflection and dialogues with other. In this last chapter synthesizing the preceding chapters in this volume, we aim to contribute to new imaginaries of society, particularly a *caring* society where evaluators not only critically question but also nurture sociopolitical practices of care when evaluating policy and programs.

CARE AS AN UNFOLDING PRAXIS

Evaluators ascribe value to policies or programs. The authors in this volume approach these policies or programs as practices that have particular histories, are infused with moral values, and have an unfolding nature. For example, teaching is a caring practice because teachers care for children's well-being and future (Van Manen & Shuying, 2002). Evaluators who work for a caring society approach practices, such as teaching, by seeing the evaluation itself as an unfolding praxis of care. These evaluators aim to understand what matters according to the people involved in these practices through an intricate process of action, reflection, and dialogue that fosters mutual understanding.

Along with the authors in this volume, we illustrate the view of evaluation as a sociopolitical activity intended to implement policies and practices that balance stakeholders' concerns. These concerns are directed to "maintaining and repairing life-sustaining webs" in evaluation settings (Fisher &

Tronto, 1990, p. 40). The evaluators in this volume critically inquire into the macro sociopolitical issues of policies, programs, and institutions while exhibiting micro-attentiveness and responsiveness to the specific other. An evaluation practice attentive in a moral sense recognizes the distinct situations of people in the context of the whole: society. Rather than making general abstractions, the evaluations in this volume are grounded in and engage with the richness and ambiguities of particular cases. This approach entails a receptiveness, responsiveness, and attentiveness to the everyday challenges and concerns of the people who constitute these practices. These are to what the evaluator can be oriented and what a care perspective on society can be about: attentiveness, responsibility, and responsiveness to foster solidarity and trust (Tronto, 2013).

In our evaluation work, *praxis* denotes a particular way of action that is not instrumental or rational (this action leads to that outcome) but morally informed, wise, prudent, and embedded in the traditions of action, reflection, and dialogue on theory and practice. Praxis focuses on "a particular kind of human engagement that involves one's dealings with, or interactions with, others that *unfolds* in view of some particular understanding of substantive rationality appropriate to the practice in question" (Schwandt, 2005, p. 98). We stress the word *unfold* in italics because it illustrates that we cannot steer or control human engagement or understanding through a rational (evidence-based) approach. We can learn from evidence, but it is impossible to simply transfer evidence gathered in one context to another. Eliot Eisner (1998) pleas for evaluators to be connoisseurs: using their sensitivities and experiences to examine the evaluand at hand.

Care ethics also favors the local and particular and rejects the universal and generalizable (Vosman & Niemeijer, 2017). Every praxis—whether professional such as teaching or personal such as cooking a meal—requires the participants' knowledge, specifically, their *phronesis* (practical wisdom) and wise judgment. Evaluators do not focus on pinpointing causal mechanisms of practices to evaluate hypotheses about effectiveness but, rather, help "practitioners understand the kinds of evaluative decisions they face and enhance their ability to deliberate well" (Schwandt, 2005, p. 99). Evaluation from a caring perspective, therefore, enhances the personal and mutual understandings of those whose lives or work is at stake. These enriched personal and mutual understandings form the basis for local action and preserve or nurture life-sustaining webs.

As a way of understanding and knowing (Eikeland, 2012), praxis then is an affective, moral, existential, material, social, embodied, and political doing that is always unfolding. From this perspective, the people involved are neither fully autonomous individuals acting at will, confronting each other with their decisions nor judgmental dopes conforming to social norms but agents who "carry" practices in their bodily and mental routines; they are agents who consist in the performance of practices. (Reckwitz, 2002, as cited in Schwandt, 2005, p. 100). Discussing the meaning of practices[2] in evaluation, Schwandt (2005) states that

> although it is undeniable that scientific information can be valuable to practices of all kinds, the kind of knowledge we seek in improving practice is not fundamentally knowledge of fact or knowledge in the form of new theories or new models for practice, nor is it only craft knowledge. There is more to "knowing" in practice than *knowing that* or *knowing how*. Rather, practice changes as practitioners change their sensibilities and sensitivities, their ways of being toward a situation. (p. 100, emphasis in original)

We want to define this kind of knowing: *knowing from within*. It is *pathic* (Van Manen & Shuying, 2002) and includes feelings and emotions, such as empathy and compassion. Evaluators for a caring society develop knowing from within through engagement with people whose lives or work is at stake, instead of retrieving knowledge from practice.

This view of evaluation also includes the unfolding of these ways of knowing and being in the context of the physical space of practices, in other words, nonhuman entities. Material realities, such as walls, are part of our world and practices, but we human beings cannot go through a wall. If we want to get to the other side of the wall, we have to walk around it or tear it down. In this volume, Freeman discusses the meaning of materialism for evaluation, particularly the meaning of new materialist and posthumanistic theory for evaluation. The issue of meaning is also addressed in the case of telecare by Pols in Chapter 5. Despite extensive publications on care from an inclusive, relational, and political perspective, including performative approaches to care (i.e., Hamington, Chapter 1), there seems to be little interest (yet) in posthumanist perspectives on care and evaluation. A posthumanist perspective would explore evaluation for a caring society as a (be)coming together of evaluative people and materials (e.g., buildings and spaces) and other living beings (e.g., plants and animals; Kunneman, 2017). Viewing society as a collective of these kinds of practices means that we can no longer steer or control this process of unfolding. Instead, we can learn how to relate and respond, listen, and be attentive to what gradually unfolds.

PEOPLE AS EVALUATIVE BEINGS

In addition to holding a praxis view of evaluation, evaluators who foster care in society honor people as evaluative beings. This means that they do not restrict evaluation to scholars or professionals but open up the activity to open to each and every person. Evaluation is a fundamental human activity. When we have a drink, we judge whether it is tasty. This is an informal evaluation of its quality. In retrospect, we may think about the criteria for why we find it tasty, but this is a rationalization. We do not need criteria to immediately sense tastiness, and we often find it hard to describe this experience. Evaluators formalize processes of quality assessment by using predetermined criteria, standards, and principles. Many evaluators, though not those in this volume, work from a principalist stance on standards based on theories such as utilitarianism and consequentialism which argue for a non-contextual definition of what is good and bad. It is assumed that standards to judge the quality of a particular program or policy can be determined in advance by the service users or the sponsors of programs and policies.

The evaluators in this volume take a different stance. In general, they carry out evaluations with the goal of deeply understanding what matters to people in the everyday situations of policy-based programs, institutions, or social practices, the value commitments they hold and enact in practice. These evaluators do not so much assess or measure—although these can be part of their work—but negotiate what is necessary and valuable for these programs, policies, and practices to grow and flourish from the perspectives of the people, the participants themselves. These evaluations give priority to including the voices of as many participants as possible.3 Such evaluations not only depart from the notion that people evaluate differently—that they are normative beings—but are also carried out with a normative purpose and approach themselves: the thought that practices can or should or could be in a certain way. These evaluations have a normative horizon: to engender a caring society which holds caring as a core value.

The everyday practices of evaluation can be seen as collectives of "evaluative beings," to use sociologist's Andrew Sayer's (2011, p. 1) words. Evaluative beings are relational, interdependent, moral, rational, affective, capable, and vulnerable. They can simultaneously experience various states of well-being and suffering and often a myriad of values are at stake in the practice under consideration. Due to their complexity, these practices often cannot be reduced to a small set of criteria or principles. Refugee children (as discussed in Chapter 4 by Hanberger) can enjoy playing with their peers and experience a sense of belonging and being cared for by their caregivers even while separation from their parents produces tremendous emotional distress. In Sayer's words, our "relation to the world is one of concern or care" (2011, p. 9). This is a normative social practice because we are continuously exploring questions such as, "What shall I do for the best?"

Evaluators who foster a caring society aim to gain insight into the moral goods embedded in practices (later, we discuss that in our work, we prefer to focus on the concepts of issues and concerns instead of criteria and standards). In responsive and democratic approaches to evaluation—those highlighted in this volume—these criteria and standards are the outcomes of a highly complex participatory process of dialogue and negotiation among the people who are part of a certain practice and hold various positions, from precarious positions to those the evaluation process strengthens. It is often difficult to pinpoint what makes a practice morally good, what the right criterion to assess its goodness are. Often, these are imposed externally, possibly resulting in a mismatch between the moral goods (tacitly) present in a particular practice.

We thus view evaluation practices as expressive collaborative (Walker, 2007) practices in which people engage with and learn about one another, and, through a process of moral learning, gain clarity on what matters to them and why. The evaluator facilitates this process. In this view, we leave behind the concept of criterion or standard as seen from a spectator's view. Here, a spectator's view refers to describing, explaining, or judging situations from a detached perspective from above. Evaluation for a caring society is embedded *within* and emerges *from* practices. It focuses not on what should or ought to be done in certain practices from a reductive point of view but, instead, moves toward personal accounts of what matters in everyday situations, why they matter to people, what the underlying value commitments entail, and what moral goods emerge. The evaluation approaches and stories in this volume illustrate how the emergence of insights in "what matters" according to participants works in everyday situations. This seems to be in line with a general trend among evaluators, care ethicists, and qualitative inquirers in general searching for ways to work with the plurality and diversity of values in practices. They all recognize multiple sources of valuation and respect the plurality of values held by people. Evaluators create communicative spaces and dialogue to articulate the emerging goods important to those whose lives and work are involved in the practice.

COMPETENCES AND INTUITIONS

The facilitation of communicative, dialogic space asks for the cultivation of particular competences and reflections on moral intuitions. The evaluator does not understand in isolation but belongs to a praxis of care while carrying out evaluations. In Chapter 1, Hamington discusses the required competencies: "Competency is not simply a technical professionalism but also entails emotional intelligence, responsiveness, and inquiry—all elements of care." Emotional competence is an important requirement to foster a practice of understanding lifeworlds, as Dahlberg demonstrates in Chapter 2. Baur, Nistelrooij, and van Vanlaere (2017) discuss the connection between emotions and care in the context of transformative research and health care professionalism. Along with other care ethicists such as Engster and Hamington (2015) and Noddings (1984), they address the connectedness of morality and emotions, arguing that emotions are a source of moral action. According to Baur, Nistelrooij, & van Vanlaere, (2017) for emotions to be productive in caring institutions, the creation of a moral space that acknowledges the presence of emotions is necessary. We believe that evaluators can cultivate this moral space by reflecting on their emotions.

Reflection on moral intuitions is also part of the reflexive practice of evaluators who aim to foster care, humanization, and moral spaces (Visse, 2012). Noddings (1984) locates the offspring of ethical behavior in human affective processes that we argue might best be labelled moral intuitions. We do not see intuitions as opposed to rational or emotional views on morality. Rather, these processes are closely interwoven and constitute a continuum (Dellantonio & Job, 2012). In our evaluations, intuitions come to the surface as we sense that something is not quite right. This can be either a bodily sensation (e.g., a faster heartbeat) or a rational or psychological sensation (e.g., a general felt sense). Intuitions here can be seen as prereflexive, embodied signs that steer the evaluation and help us to articulate what matters. Evaluators who aim to establish a caring society, moreover, should reflect on their own processes of over- and under-identification to reduce bias and promote moral openness, which are necessary for an open moral space (Visse, Abma, & Widdershoven, 2012; Walker, 2007). This entails a critical analysis of one's own social (privileged) positions, assumptions, prejudices, and preferences in moral relations and evaluator identities (Visse et al., 2012; Walker, 2007).

DIALOGUE AND REFLECTION

Consequently and fundamentally, an important aim of evaluators working for a caring society is to view practices as a coming together of people who enter a reflexive dialogue on what matters to them in a particular program or policy. The dialogue is considered to be an open space for personal and mutual learning and reflection with the purpose of reaching mutual understandings. In contrast to a persuasive dialogue, this type of dialogue builds on reflection and the willingness to pause in a conversation and to spend time and explore more deeply what seems to be essential to the participants. Dialogue and reflection are simultaneously appreciative and critical. Before genuine dialogue is possible, the participants need to have a sense of safety and trust. The evaluator acts as a process facilitator creating the conditions for a genuine dialogue among different persons who share their personal stories. They are open to sharing only in a space of trust and mutual respect. Once these requirements are met, a more critical approach can be taken, questioning one's assumptions and differences on the topic. Reflection occurs not outside the evaluation practice but in line with Karen Barad's (2007) concept of diffraction, which attends and responds "to the effects of difference" (Barad, 2007, p. 72) and examines the "entanglements" that differences make (Barad, 2007, p. 73). An evaluator who follows a diffractive approach to reflexivity is part of the world evaluated and does not occupy a spectator position. Chapter 8 describes what this means in practice.

We acknowledge that knowledge and knowing can only be partial. Several authors in this volume address the practice and acceptance of not-knowing as important to fostering care through evaluation. Dahlberg (Chapter 2) frames this not-knowing as a cornerstone of caring, a prerequisite for listening and seeing the lifeworld of another. Bos and Abma (Chapter 7) speak about unknowable otherness and claim that it demands that we respond to it with moral humility and a passible performance. They refer to the work of Bernard Waldenfels (2004), who understands otherness as relational; the other is unfamiliar and strange to us as long as we insert our own frames of reference into the middle of knowing (logocentrism) and cannot deal with aspects that do not fit. We either romanticize the other as exotic or see the other as a variation of ourselves. It is difficult not to reduce the other's perspective to something we are able to understand, because to avoid doing so, we have to mistrust and bypass mainstream (or culturally accepted) knowledge and knowledge production processes. Alternative shared-knowledge construction work is a risky and sometimes violent endeavour, requiring critical reflexivity. How do we get to know a person who hardly speaks and has multiple disabilities? Bos and Abma (Chapter 7) show that in this instance, we cannot rely on the dia-logos with which we are familiar and have to enter a new relational-experiential space. They suggest that prolonged familiarization with the context helps develop a way of knowing that better does justice to the non-verbality of persons with intellectual disabilities.

Many authors in this volume focus on creating spaces where people can learn about their experiences by sharing their stories. This process of mutual learning generates a dialogic understanding of a caring society that has still space for ambiguity, uncertainty and—to quote our care ethical colleagues Vosman and Niemeijer (2017)—precariousness.

OPENNESS AS AN ISSUE AND CONCERN FOR CONCEPTUAL ORGANIZERS

In our work, issues and concerns are the conceptual organizers for evaluations, rather than needs, objectives, hypotheses, social and economic equations (Stake, 1995), and other standardized criteria imposed by external system requirements, such as productivity, safety, and efficiency. Problematically, these top-down, externally imposed criteria rarely are meaningful to the practices they concern. Moreover, these system values undermine the moral values inherent to caring practices, thereby undermining practitioners' morale and moral identity (Abma, Leyerzapf, & Landeweer, 2016). The issues and concerns embedded within and derived from the practice relate to the interactivity, particularity, and subjective and sensory valuing already felt by the persons associated with a policy or program. They are concerned (or likely to become concerned) about certain matters, and the evaluators inquire, negotiate, and select several issues and concerns around which to organize the study. As Abma (2005; Greene & Abma, 2001) suggests, this selection of issues should be a joint affair to ensure that they are meaningful to all involved and relevant to the local context. Often, these issues and concerns are multi-layered, morally complex, and controversial, raising debate and discussion among the people involved and within the practice under consideration (Abma & Noordegraaf, 2003; Abma, Voskes, & Widdershoven, 2017).

Starting from the issues and concerns in the practice is closely linked to the work of care ethicists who use theoretical concepts such as precariousness as heuristic concepts or critical insights that function as lenses to observe the moral good in particular practices (Leget, van Nistelrooij, & Visse, 2017; Vosman & Niemeijer, 2017). We thus open ourselves to wonderment about what matters to others (Hansen, 2012). In evaluation studies such as those in this volume, the issues and concerns of the evaluands direct the evaluation process. Often, these issues and concerns are tacitly present in people's stories and doings. Most evaluators in this volume put the actual personal stories of people at the center of evaluation. The evaluators temporarily become part of these practices through participatory work, such as having conversations, doing participant observations, shadowing participants, reconstructing stories, and dialoguing about their texts. During these evaluation activities, the evaluators honor a pluralistic, particular view on merit to meet individuals' concerns. They know how to wonder (Hansen, 2012) about the complexities of the lifeworlds and the lived (bodily) experiences of the people in the practices. Evaluations tell multiple stories integrating the lived experiences and interpretations of people regarding policy (Abma, 1999, 2000), programs, and institutions into a multi-fractured whole. This whole is not necessarily coherent or unambiguous but produces fuller, thicker descriptions and literary texts than more traditional ways of reporting in the social sciences.

DIGNITY

In Chapter 3, Greene and Simons explicitly address the value of advancing dignity in their approach to democratic evaluation. The care ethics field has a body of work on dignity (Leget, 2013; Sayer 2011). Rather than viewing dignity primarily as the property of a person from which abstract, inalienable rights can be derived, dignity is informed and refined by critical insights from daily (policy) practice(s). Dignity appears to be "an intersubjective category which is constituted and upheld by people who are interrelated in caring relationships" (Leget, 2013, p. 955) and closely related to vulnerability, fragility and well being (Sayer, 2011).

Leget (2013) formulates three questions to explore dignity from which evaluators can benefit. Firstly, the evaluator can assess how vulnerable people feel or experience dignity in the evaluation context (Leget [2013], in the context of health care, formulates this question as follows: "What is the meaning of the concept of dignity as used by patients who express their subjective experiences?"). This can provide the evaluator with insight into stakeholders' complex, often ambiguous lifeworlds. Leget (2013) argues for a phenomenological and hermeneutical approach that we believe can profoundly deepen the work of evaluators. Second, this care ethical view on dignity can inspire evaluators to ask social-relational questions on dignity: What is the quality of the relations in the evaluation as seen from the perspectives of several stakeholders, such as the perspectives of professionals, patients, family members, and volunteers? Third, Leget (2013) addresses dignity in the sociopolitical context: What is a person's social position? This concerns a person's collective position or belonging to a sociopolitical and cultural group. This care ethical approach to human dignity was developed with the participation by different stakeholders and although it is not applied out in a formal evaluation study, this work builds on other participatory approaches to understand and foster care. Further studies could explore how dignity is conceptualized and practiced in everyday policies and programs.

PLURALISM, POWER, AND PRECARIOUSNESS

Another element of evaluation for a caring society is to recognize and actively work with power and asymmetric relations. The evaluation literature and this volume give ample examples of what this entails. The chapters in Part IV report on evaluations in highly political, power-laden social contexts. Asymmetric relations and issues of power are present everywhere, including less politically charged settings. Subtle differences in power, sometimes enacted as micro-aggressions (Leyerzapf et al., Chapter 9), are harder to notice but do not have less importance to or influence on evaluands' practices. Again, bodily sensations, such a faster heartbeat or sweaty hands, can inform us about imbalances in power rather well, but evaluations often neglect these. Evaluators should be attentive and responsive to these differences in power and develop their competencies to work constructively with differences (Baur, Van Elteren, Nierse, & Abma, 2010; Visse et al., 2015).

In addition, evaluators can learn from care ethicists by rethinking power in the context of late-modern society (Vosman & Niemeijer, 2017). Vosman and Niemeijer (2017) offer a perspective that moves beyond seeing power as oppression toward a view of power based on notions of precariousness and uncertainty. Precariousness is seen as powerlessness against insecurity (Vosman & Niemeijer, 2017, p. 8). What occurs when evaluators put precariousness at the center of their work? Responsiveness to plurality stresses the political features of evaluation practices and the presence of asymmetries in relationships. However, instead of seeing asymmetries and power as opposing factors, care ethicists view asymmetry and power as "a centripetal force, a foundation for relations of domination and submission" (Nistelrooij, 2014, p. 39). This is not the suppression of one group of people by another (e.g., not including their voices) "but the more subtle working of power [that] spreads insecurity that can engulf the lives of many, the seemingly dominant people as well" (Vosman & Niemeijer, 2017, p. 10). In several chapters, we can see that people on the margin are not intentionally marginalized, but certain caring arrangements reestablish structural inequalities and discrimination because taken-for-granted norms, such as heteronormativity, Whiteness, and ableism, drive and normalize practices.

Attending to pluralism when evaluating for a caring society also means explicitly acknowledging differences in gender, race, and sexuality (chapters in Part IV). To deepen our understanding of these dimensions, we recommend that evaluators explore the promises of an intersectional approach to evaluation. Intersectionality is close to our approach because it focuses on the meaning and consequences of interactive and interlocking social relations, power structures, and processes without dividing differences into social categories such as "race, class, or gender" (Hankivsky, 2014, p. 253). Instead, intersectionality views social practices from a critical intersectional perspective on established power relations in society (Verdonk, Muntinga, Leyerzapf, & Abma, 2017; McCall 2005).

DIFFERENCES BETWEEN CONTINENTS

> Consider yourself to be a scientist in the early forties—what to think of European ideas and science in a part of the world where fascism, Nazism were taking root? It was not until the sixties, when immigrants from Germany and other parts of Europe had settled in America, and the time was such that people got very interested in politics that Continental philosophers were included. Important figures are C. Wright Mills and Gouldner. They acknowledged that values are part of knowing. So it is part of the history of American social science that values were not taken into account. I think Weberian ideas about "wert-frei" science also have had a great impact on social science. (Schwandt, personal communication, Summer 1994)

In this personal communication with one of us (Tineke), Tom Schwandt sketches the backdrop of continental differences in the evaluation discipline and profession. This helps us understand that evaluation in the United States, as part of North American social science initially ignored the value-ladenness of its practice even though the discipline encompassed valuing. Schwandt's teacher, Egon Guba (personal communication, 1994), recalls that he gave a lecture on a-experimental designs in 1966 and was told to bury the paper because it might undermine his career. He did so successfully, in his words: "I repressed it so successfully that for 15 years I couldn't remember that I had done it. Till someone reminded me and asked me for a copy, I replied, 'What paper?'" (Guba, personal communication).

The field of evaluation has developed and changed tremendously since then. The field of care ethics dates to Sara Ruddick's (1980) essay "*Maternal Thinking*," Carol Gilligan's (1982) "*In a Different Voice*," and Nel Nodding's (1984) *Caring: A Feminine Approach to Ethics and Moral Education.* Care ethics was a response to and critique on dominant values like justice and autonomy, and 'moral boundaries' between the private and public domain that kept gendered social hierarchies in place and devalued care work to the private domain (Tronto, 1993). Like evaluation studies, it is a growing rapidly field, and scholars from a rich variety of disciplines contribute to and are inspired by its development (e.g., Bourgault, 2016; Conradi & Vosman, 2016; Engster & Hamington, 2015; Leget et al., 2017; Tronto, 2013, 2010; Zembylas, Bozalek, & Shefer, 2014). Until now, we only know of ample evaluators who integrate a care approach into their work, but we believe this field is expanding globally. In this volume, Greene and Simons explicitly address differences in European and American evaluation approaches. They point out that context matters, especially in a field where cultural and sociopolitical developments, institutional arrangements, and intellectual traditions heavily influence the subject of evaluation (policies and programs).

Worth mentioning here is one period in the intellectual history of evaluation which inspired many of those on whose shoulders we stand and demonstrates the power of international intellectual cooperation (Abma, 1994, 1998; Abma & Widdershoven, 2000). It goes back to the mid-1960s, when in the United States, Lee Cronbach proposed that the evaluation field needed good social anthropologists. This call inspired many evaluators to become naturalistic or field researchers with a special focus on lived experiences and social relations (Stake, 1991; personal communication, summer 1994). On the other side of the Atlantic Ocean, at the United Kingdom's Center for Applied Research (CARE), Malcolm Parlett and David Hamilton (1972) elaborated the metaphor of the evaluator as social anthropologist. They proposed an illuminative approach to evaluation that is adaptable to situations. Central to this approach, evaluators familiarize themselves "thoroughly with the day-to-day reality... to unravel the complexity" (Parlett & Hamilton, 1972).

During this lively period, Barry MacDonald (1977), discussed in this volume by Simons and Greene, developed his democratic approach to evaluation, along with an overseas network between CARE and the Center for Instructional Research and Curriculum Evaluation (CIRCE) in the United States. At CIRCE, Stake (1967; Abma & Stake, 2001) also proposed a broader conceptualization of evaluation that included social interactions. Evaluators should not only gather data about program input and outcomes but also describe the context and judge the quality of intermediary processes. Guba and Lincoln (1989) refer explicitly to Stake's work in developing their naturalistic approach to evaluation and later the Fourth Generation Evaluation (Guba & Lincoln, 1989).

Similarly, there are commonalities and differences in the practice of care and evaluation in the Scandinavian countries (Sweden, Chapters 2 and 4), the United Kingdom (Chapter 3), Germany (Chapter 6), and the Netherlands (Part IV). Rapid growth always raises the risk of reducing a complex field into an instrumental application of care or evaluation. We, therefore, argue for a slow, careful approach to exploring this interesting intersection of two fields.

IMAGINE A CARING SOCIETY

Without an explicit discussion, this volume gives rich visions of how a caring society could look like and be imagined and the role of evaluation. In between its lines, this book breathes an evaluation imaginary (Schwandt, 2009) and a social imaginary (Taylor, 2004). The evaluation imaginary is not the image of evaluation as an audit or assessment culture (Dahler-Larssen, 2012, p. 99). Instead—just like the image of a caring society—it is about dialogue, reflection, openness, plurality, materiality, inclusion, respect for difference, and working with moral-political and creative dimensions in everyday practices. In its own way, evaluation *is* a practice of care.

To conclude, imagination has and still plays a central role in our dialogical work through the use of artistic approaches to understand care (Visse, 2017), the application of narrative and poetic vignettes (Visse, 2017; Visse et al., 2012) and the organization and facilitation of narrative workshops (Abma, 2003; Abma & Widdershoven, 2008). If we, as a community of evaluators and care ethicists, aim to foster a caring society, we will advocate for more attention to the intersection of creativity, ethics, and evaluation. Inspired by evaluation theorists such as Tom Schwandt and Peter Dahler-Larsen, moral philosophy scholars such as John Wall (2005) and Charlotte Dixon & Helen Haste (2014), and activists such as Sara Ahmed (2017) and

Rebecca Solnit (2016), we will go further explore the promises of social imaginaries and creativity in the context of evaluation and care (Dahler-Larsen, 2012; Dixon & Haste, 2014; Schwandt, 2009; Wall, 2005).

Sara Ahmed (2017) calls for us to develop our imagination through *sweaty concepts* (as opposed to dry abstractions) which emerge from the shattering phenomenological experience of changing practices, "finding ways to keep going, to keep trying, even when the same things happen to us over and over again" (Ahmed, 2017, p. 163). Rebecca Solnit (2016) reminds us that hope of a better future is open, or to quote Virginia Woolf, the future is dark, not in the sense of blackness or pessimism but in the sense of open-mindedness, unknown, and unknowable. Finally, Kenneth Gergen and Mary Gergen (2012) inspire us to develop notions of "what could be" (versus "what is") through performance art (p. 29). This can be a liberating experience:

> The fact that science could change the world by studying it was viewed as a fatal flaw in positivist research; for constructionists, it represents a major opportunity. From the charting of "what is," the role of science becomes that of creating "what could be." (Gergen & Gergen, 2012, p. 31)

We hope that this volume and synthesis can serve as a guide or even an ethos for evaluators who aim for a caring society. This synthesis clarifies that to us, evaluation for a caring society is not a scientific endeavor but a moral-political praxis. Evaluators acknowledge this praxis, including its richness and complexity, during the ongoing process of dialogue and reflection. When carrying out evaluations, whether in health care, public administration, education, or environmental policies, we together we learn what a caring society can be as we imagine what it can become.

NOTES

1. Visse and Niemeijer (2016; Niemeijer & Visse, 2016) explored inquiry as a praxis of care in their publications on relational ethnography.
2. Practice as in rehearsing, training, or mastery is not praxis. Eikeland (2012) clearly describes the differences.
3. The evaluation literature thoroughly discuss the complexities and considerations in the decision-making process about whose voices to include and exclude because including all voices all the time is not possible (e.g., Abma, 2006; Greene, 2000).

REFERENCES

Abma, T. A. (1994). *Responsive evaluation: In conversation with its creators.* [Personal communication]. Rotterdam, Netherlands: Institute for Health Care Policy and management, Erasmus University.

Abma, T. A. (1998). Writing for dialogue: Text in evaluation context. *Evaluation, 4*(4), 434–454.

Abma, T. A. (Ed.). (1999). *Telling tales on narrative and evaluation.* Stamford, CT: JAI Press/Ablex Publishing Corporation.

Abma, T. A. (2000). Fostering learning-in-organizing through narration: Questioning myths and stimulating multiplicity in two performing art schools. *European Journal of Work & Organization Psychology, 9*(2), 211–232.

Abma, T. (2003). Learning by telling: Storytelling workshops as an organizational learning intervention. *Management Learning, 34*(2), 221–240.

Abma, T. A. (2005). The practice and politics of responsive evaluation. *American Journal of Evaluation, 27*(1), 31–43.

Abma, T. (2006). The practice and politics of responsive evaluation. *American Journal of Evaluation, 27*(1), 31–43.

Abma, T. A., & Noordegraaf, M. (2003). Managers amidst ambiguity. Towards a typology of evaluative practices in management settings. *Evaluation, 9*(3), 285–306.

Abma, T. A., & Widdershoven, G. A. M. (2011). Evaluation as a relationally responsive practice. In N. Denzin & Y. S. Lincoln (Eds.), *Qualitative research. SAGE handbook* (pp. 669–680). Los Angeles, CA: SAGE.

Abma, T., & Widdershoven, G. (2008). Evaluation as social relation. *Evaluation, 14*(2), 209–225.

Abma, T., Voskes, Y., & Widdershoven, G. (2017). Participatory bioethics research and its social impact: The case of coercion reduction in psychiatry. *Bioethics, 31*(2), 144–152.

Abma, T. A. H., Leyerzapf, E., & Landeweer, E. (2016). Responsive evaluation in the Interference zone between system and lifeworld. *American Journal of Evaluation,* 1–14. doi:10.1177/1098214016667211

Ahmed, S. (2017). *Living a feminist life.* Durham, NC: Duke University Press.

Barad, K. (2007). *Meeting the universe halfway: Quantum physics and the entanglement of matter and meaning.* Durham, NC: Duke University Press.

Baur, V. E., Van Elteren, A. H. G., Nierse, C. J., & Abma, T. A. (2010). Dealing with distrust and power dynamics: Asymmetric relations among stakeholders in responsive evaluation. *Evaluation, 16*(3), 233–248.

Baur, V., Nistelrooij, I., & van Vanlaere, L. (2017). The sensible health care professional: A care ethical perspective on the role of caregivers in emotionally turbulent practices. *Medicine, Healthcare and Philosophy.* doi:10.1007/s11019-017-9770-5

Bourgault, S. (2016). Prolegomena to a caring bureaucracy. *European Journal of Women's Studies, (24)*3, 202–217.

Conradi, E., & Vosman, F. (2016). *Praxis der Achtsamkeit. Schlüsselbegriffe der Care-Ethik* [Praxis of Care: Key Insights of Care Ethics]. Frankfurt am Main, Germany: Campus Verlag.

Dahler-Larsen, P. (2012). *The evaluation society.* Stanford, CA: Stanford University Press.

Dellantonio, S., & Job, R. (2012). Moral intuitions vs. moral reasoning. A philosophical analysis of the explanatory models intuitionism relies on. In L. Magnani & P. Li (Eds.), *Philosophy and cognitive science. Studies in applied philosophy, epistemology and rational ethics* (Vol. 2, pp. 239–262). Berlin, Germany: Springer.

Dixon, C., & Haste, H. (2014). The dialogic witness: New metaphors of creative and ethical work. In S. Moran, J. C. Kaufman, & D. Cropley (Eds.), *The ethics of creativity* (pp. 232–239). Basingstoke, England: Palgrave Macmillan.

Eikeland, O. (2012). Action research-applied research, intervention research, collaborative research, practitioner research, or praxis *research? International Journal of Action Research, 8*(1), 9–44.

Eisner, E. W. (1998). *The enlightened eye: qualitative inquiry and the enhancement of educational practice.* Upper Saddle River, NJ: Merrill.

Engster, D., & Hamington, M. (2015). *Care ethics & political theory.* Oxford, England: Oxford University Press.

Fisher, B., & Tronto, J. (1990). Toward a feminist theory of caring. In E. Abel & M. Nelson (Eds.), *Circles of care* (pp. 36–54). Albany: State University of New York Press.

Gergen, K., & Gergen, M. (2012). *Playing with purpose.* Walnut Creek, CA: Left Coast Press.

Gilligan, C. (1982). *In a different voice.* Boston, MA: Harvard University Press.

Greene, J. (2000). Challenges in practicing deliberative democratic evaluation. *New Directions for Evaluation, 85,* 13–26.

Greene, J. C., & Abma, T. A. (Eds.). (2001). Responsive evaluation. *New Directions for Evaluation,* 92.

Guba, E., Lincoln, G. (1989). Fourth Generation Evaluation. Beverly Hills, CA: SAGE.

Hankivsky, O. (2014). Rethinking care ethics: On the promise and potential of an intersectional analysis. *American Political Science Review, 108*(2), 252–264.

Hansen, F. T. (2012). One step further: The dance between poetic dwelling and Socratic wonder in phenomenological research. *Indo-Pacific Journal of Phenomenology, 12,* 1–20.

Kittay, E. F. (1999). *Love's labor: Essays on women, equality and dependency.* New York, NY: Routledge.

Kunneman, H. (2017, October 5). *Radical humanism.* Afscheidsrede, University of Humanistic Studies, Utrecht, Netherlands.

Leget, C. (2013). Analyzing dignity: A perspective from the ethics of care. *Medicine, Health Care and Philosophy, 16*(4), 945–52

Leget, C., van Nistelrooij, I., & Visse, M. (2017). Beyond demarcation: Care ethics as an interdisciplinary field of enquiry. *Nursing Ethics.* doi:0969733017707008

MacDonald, B. (1977). A political classification of evaluation studies. In D. Hamilton, D. *numbers game* (pp. 224–227). London, England: Macmillan.

McCall, L. (2005). The complexity of intersectionality. *SIGNS: Journal of Women in Culture and Society, 30*(31), 1771–802.

Niemeijer, A., & Visse, M. A. (2016). Challenging standard concepts of 'humane' care through relational auto-ethnography. *Inclusion, 4*(4):168–175.

Nistelrooij, I. (2014). *Sacrifice: A care-ethical reappraisal of sacrifice and self-sacrifice.* (Doctoral dissertation). University of Humanistic Studies, Utrecht, Netherlands).

Noddings, N. (1984). *Caring: A feminine approach to ethics and moral education.* Berkeley, CA: University of California Press.

Parlett, M., & Hamilton, D. (1972). Evaluation as illumination: A new approach to the study of innovatory programs. In G. Glass (Ed.), *Evaluation review studies annual* (Vol. 1, pp. 140–157). Beverly Hills, CA: SAGE.

Ruddick, S. (1980). Maternal Thinking. *Feminist Studies, 6*(2), 342.

Sayer, A. (2011). *Why things matter to people. Social science, values and ethical life.* New York, NY, Cambridge University Press.

Schön, D. A. (1991). *The reflective practitioner: How professionals think in action.* Aldershot, England: Ashgate.

Schwandt, T. (2009). Globalization influences on the Western evaluation imaginary. In K. E. Ryan & B. J. Cousins (Eds.), *Sage international handbook of educational evaluation* (pp. 19–36). Thousand Oaks, CA: SAGE.

Schwandt, T. S. (2005). On modeling our understanding of the practice fields. *Pedagogy, Culture and Society, 13*(3), 313–332.

Solnit, R. (2016). *Hope in the dark, untold histories, wild possibilities.* London, England: Canongate.

Stake, R. E. (1967). The countenance of evaluation. *Teachers College Record, 68,* 523–540.

Stake, R. (1991). Responsive evaluation and qualitative methods. In W. Shadish, T. Cook, & L. Leviton (Eds.), *Foundations of program evaluation* (pp. 270–314). Thousand Oaks, CA: SAGE.

Stake, R. (1995). *The art of case study research.* Thousand Oaks, CA: SAGE.

Tronto, J. (2010). Creating caring institutions: Politics, plurality and process. *Ethics and Social Welfare, 4*(2), 158–171.

Tronto, J. (2013). *Caring democracy. Markets, equality and justice.* New York, NY: New York University Press.

Van Manen, M., & Shuying, L. (2002). The pathic principle of pedagogical language. *Teaching and Teacher Education, 18*(2), pp. 215–224.

Verdonk, P., Muntinga, M. E., Leyerzapf, H., & Abma, T. A. (forthcoming). Strategic reciprocation between condensed categories and fluid identities. Understanding and studying dynamic differences in healthcare from an intersectional perspective. In *Bringing intersectionality to public policy.*

Visse, M. (2017). Nested tensions in care. *American Medical Association: Journal of Ethics, 19*(4), 399–405.

Visse, M. A. (2012). *Openings for humanization in modern health care practices.* (PhD dissertation). Amsterdam, VU University Amsterdam.

Visse, M. A., Abma, T. A., & Widdershoven, G. A. M. (2012). Relational responsibilities in responsive evaluation. *Evaluation and Program Planning, 35,* 97–104.

Visse, M. A., Abma, T. A., & Widdershoven, G. A. M. (2015). Practising political care ethics: Can responsive evaluation foster democratic care? *Ethics & Social Welfare, 9*(2), 164–182.

Visse, M., & Niemeijer, A. (2016). Autoethnography as a praxis of care: The promises of (political) autoethnograhpy as an epistemology and method. *International Journal of Qualitative Inquiry, 16*(3), 301–312.

Vosman, F., & Niemeijer, A. (2017). Rethinking critical reflection on care: Late *Care and Philosophy*. doi: 10.1007/s11019-017-9766-1

Waldenfels, B. (2004). Bodily experience between selfhood and otherness. *Phenomenology and the Cognitive Sciences, 3*, 235–248.

Walker, M. U. (2007). *Moral understandings. A feminist study in ethics.* London, England: Routledge.

Wall, J. (2005). *Moral creativity.* New York, NY: Oxford University Press.

Zembylas, M., Bozalek, V., & Shefer, T. (2014). Tronto's notion of privileged irresponsibility and the reconceptualisation of care: Implications for critical pedagogies of emotion in higher education. *Gender and Education, 26*, 200–214. doi:10.1080/09540253.2014.901718

ABOUT THE CONTRIBUTORS

Tineke A. Abma, MSc, PhD (1964) is Full Professor Participation & Diversity and head of the Department of Medical Humanities and research leader in the Amsterdam School of Public Health, VU University Medical Center, Amsterdam. In 2010 she was appointed as an endowed chair in the field of Client Participation in Elderly care. In 2013 she received an ASPASIA laureate from NWO for excellent female researchers. She published extensively in the fields of program evaluation and qualitative research, patient participation, and care ethics. Elderly care, chronic care, disability studies, and (coercion reduction in) psychiatry are her main practice fields. Her work has been awarded for its social value impact.

Gustaaf F. Bos (1982) received his master's degree in Psychology in 2009 at the RUG University Groningen (Netherlands). Between 2010 and 2015 he conducted responsive PhD-research at the VU University Amsterdam on what happens in encounters between people with and without intellectual disabilities in "reversed integration" settings. Since 2016 he has been working at the Department of Medical Humanities from the VU University Medical Centre on participatory projects regarding participation and experiential knowledge of people with an intellectual disability. Moreover, he is involved in a pilot project that facilitates and creates encounters between people with and without a severe intellectual and/or multiple disability. The aim of this project is to make the latter more visible and to enlarge their social network.

Evaluation for a Caring Society, pages 243–246

Karin Dahlberg is a professor in health sciences, now partly retired. She has been a professor at Linnaeus University in Sweden where she developed and directed a doctoral program of health sciences as well as a center for Lifeworld Research. She has been a visiting scholar at several universities in the United States and in the United Kingdom, and has given a number of summer courses in the philosophy and methodology of phenomenology in, for example, the United States, United Kingdom, and Lithuania and she is on the editorial board for several international journals. Amongst her international publications is *Reflective Lifeworld Research* (2nd edition, 2008), Studentlitteratur (Sweden, with H. Dahlberg & M. Nyström). Her latest research has been devoted to the issue of evidence (cf. van Wijngaarden, E & van der Meide, H., & Dahlberg, K. (2017): "Researching Health Care as a Meaningful Practice: Towards a Non-Dualistic View on Evidence for Qualitative Research." *Qualitative Health Research.* doi:10.1177/1049732317711133.

Melissa Freeman is a professor of qualitative research and evaluation methodologies at the University of Georgia. Her research into philosophically-informed traditions has been to understand the variety of analytical strategies used to make sense of the world, to disrupt conventional ways of thinking about research, and to open up new trajectories for research and evaluation. Her most recent book is *Modes of Thinking for Qualitative Data Analysis* (2017).

Maurice Hamington is Executive Director of University Studies and Professor of Philosophy at Portland State University. He is the author or editor of several books on care as well as dozens of articles. His works include *Care Ethics and Political Theory* (with Daniel Engster), *Applying Care Ethics to Business* (with Maureen Sander-Staudt), *Socializing Care* (with Dorothy C. Miller), and *Embodied Care.* For more information regarding his publications, please see https://pdx.academia.edu/MauriceHamington

Helen Kohlen is Professor of Care Policy and Ethics at the Philosophical-Theological University of Vallendar (PTHV) in Germany and an adjunct professor at the University of Alberta in Edmonton, Canada. She studied social science and health care science and has a background in nursing. Her research focuses on the transformation of caring practices with a focus on end-of-life care in intensive care. She did transnational research on hospital ethics committees and designs caring committees together with clinical practitioners all over Germany. Currently, she is investigating into cultural diversity and conflicts in health care practices.

Jennifer C. Greene is a professor of educational psychology at the University of Illinois at Urbana-Champaign. Her work focuses on the intersection of social science methodology and social policy and aspires to be both methodologically innovative and socially responsible. Greene's methodological research has concentrated on advancing qualitative and mixed methods approaches to social inquiry, as well as democratic commitments in evaluation practice. She is currently co-editor for the *Evaluation and Society* series, and author of *Mixed Methods in Social Inquiry*. Greene is the past president of the American Evaluation Association.

Anders Hanberger is professor of evaluation at Umea University, Sweden. He has published articles on democratic evaluation, the evaluation of public policies and programs, evaluation systems, the interplay between evaluation and governance, and evaluation methodology. He has evaluated national and local programs in various policy sectors, including social work, where, for example, he has examined programs targeting unaccompanied children and victims of honor-related violence. Special interests are the role of evaluation in democracy, the interplay between democracy and evaluation, and the consequences and constitutive effects of evaluation.

Hannah Leyerzapf, MA Cultural Anthropology, is a researcher and teacher at the Department of Medical Humanities VUmc. She conducted research on participation, empowerment, diversity, and inclusion in different care contexts. Her PhD focuses on cultural diversity of professionals in academic medicine and health care, considering intersections with ethnicity/race, gender and social class, aspects of White privilege and critical diversity management, and organizational change.

Jeannette Pols is Socrates Professor of Social Theory, Humanism, and Materialities, in the Department of Anthropology and the Health, Care, and the Body Program of the University of Amsterdam. She is also an associate professor and principal investigator in the Medical Ethics section of the Academic Medical Centre in Amsterdam. The core of Pols's research is empirical ethics in care, which studies "normativity in practice."

Helen Simons Professor of Evaluation and Education, at the University of Southampton. She specializes in case study, policy and program evaluation of education, health and social initiatives and has directed evaluation training in over 20 countries. One of the first to implement democratic evaluation in the UK, her evaluation practice is always guided by the political and ethical principles underpinning this approach. Helen has published widely on the theory and practice of evaluation, case study methodology democratic evaluation and evaluation ethics. Her book *Getting to Know Schools in a Democracy* was awarded an international book prize for "a most outstanding contribution to the social purposes of education." She has also played a major role nationally and internationally promoting the ethics of evaluation and research. Helen is a past president of the United Kingdom Evaluation

Society (UKES), a Fellow of the Academy of Social Sciences, UK and of the Royal Society of Arts.

Merel Visse is an associate professor of Care Ethics & Policy at the University of Humanistic Studies in the Netherlands. Since 1996, her research focuses on processes of humanization in all realms of society, especially health care and social welfare practices. She carried out a vast amount of responsive evaluations in hospital, chronic illness, and local community settings. Currently she is a coordinator of the global Care Ethics Research Consortium (www.care-ethics.org) and she is working on a 3-year program on artistic research in care, evaluation, and ethics, that is sponsored by her university and the Aspasia Grant for talented female scholars. For more information on her work: www.merelvisse.com

Printed in the United States
By Bookmasters